The End of Cancer:

Staying healthy and safe from Cancer

Tranquil Khan

Table of contents.

CHAPTER ONE

What is Cancer?

When your genes lose control over how your cells divide, cancer develops. For instance, aged cells might proliferate and create aberrant cells rather than dying.

When cells in your body divide more quickly than usual, a disorder called cancer may result. These unnatural cells develop into a mass or tumor.

One of the biggest causes of mortality worldwide is cancer. The World Health Organization (WHO) estimated that in 2020, cancer accounted for about 1 in 6 fatalities. Every day, professionals are putting innovative cancer therapies to the test.

Breast, lung, colon, rectum, and prostate cancers are the most prevalent types of cancer. The use of cigarettes, having a high body mass index, drinking alcohol, eating few fruits and vegetables, and not exercising account for around one-third of cancer-related fatalities.

In low- and lower-middle-income nations, cancer-causing infections including the human papillomavirus (HPV) and hepatitis are thought to be the cause of 30% of cancer cases.

If caught early and appropriately treated, many tumors are curable.

Any illness that may affect any region of the body is referred to as cancer. Neoplasms and malignant tumors are other words that are used. One characteristic of cancer is the rapid development of aberrant cells that expand outside of their normal borders, infiltrate other body components, and eventually move to other organs. This process is known as metastasis. The main reason why cancer patients die is because of widespread metastases.

Causes of cancer

There are several causes of cancer, some of which may be avoided.

For instance, statistics from 2014 indicate that smoking cigarettes cause approximately 480,000 deaths in the United States each year.

Risk factors for cancer, in addition to smoking, include:

- excessive alcohol use.
- additional body weight.
- active inactivity.
- unsound nutrition.

Other cancer-causing factors cannot be avoided. Age is now the most important unavoidable risk factor. The American Cancer Society reports that 87 percent of cancer diagnoses in Americans aged 50 or older are identified by physicians.

Is Cancer genetic?

The onset of cancer may be influenced by genetic factors.

The genetic coding of a person determines when their cells will divide and die. Gene changes may result in incorrect instructions, which may cause cancer.

Proteins contain many of the instructions for cellular development and division, and genes may also affect how proteins are produced by the cells.

Certain genes alter the proteins that would typically mend harmed cells. This could result in cancer. The changed instructions might be passed on to a child if a parent has these genes.

Some genetic alterations may take place after birth, and risks might be increased by things like smoking and sun exposure.

The chemical signals that control how the body uses, or "expresses," certain genes undergo other alterations that might result in cancer.

Finally, a propensity to a certain form of cancer might be inherited. This may be referred to as hereditary cancer syndrome by a doctor. The development of 5–10% of cancer patients is profoundly influenced by inherited genetic alterations.

How is cancer's stage identified?

To ascertain the degree and seriousness of your cancer, your healthcare professional will run tests. Your diagnosis will then be given a number. The greater the population, the greater the spread of the disease.

What are cancer's four stages?

Four phases are typical for malignancies. The size and location of the tumor are two of the many variables that affect the stage:

Stage I: Cancer has not progressed to the lymph nodes or other tissues and is contained in a limited location.

Stage II: Cancer has grown but not spread.

Stage III: Cancer has become bigger and could have gotten into other tissues, such as lymph nodes.

Stage IV: Cancer has spread to further organs or body parts. Additionally known as metastatic or advanced cancer, this stage.

There is stage zero in addition to the more typical phases I through IV. Cancer in this first stage is still contained in the region where it first appeared. Most healthcare professionals regard cancers that are still at stage zero to be precancerous and readily curable.

Types of cancers

The majority of individuals are aware of someone in their family who has received a cancer diagnosis. The sooner cancer is discovered by specialists, the sooner treatment may begin. Therefore, being aware of the most prevalent cancers and their symptoms is useful.

Considering factors like age, gender, and racial or ethnic group, there are more than 100 different forms of cancer, with some being more prevalent than others. (For instance, only males may get prostate cancer, although women are far more likely to develop breast cancer.)

Remember that many malignancies don't show symptoms in the beginning. You'll need testing to determine the reason if you do have symptoms since they might coexist with other illnesses.

CHAPTER TWO

1. Breast Cancer

Mutations, which are alterations in the genes that control cell development, are what lead to cancer. The cells may expand and divide uncontrollably thanks to the mutations.

Breast cancer is a kind of cancer that starts in breast tissue. Usually, breast cancer develops in the ducts or lobules of the breast.

The milk is produced by lobules, and ducts are the channels that carry it from the glands to the nipple. Additionally, cancer may develop in your breast's fatty tissue or fibrous connective tissue.

The unchecked cancer cells often spread to neighboring healthy breast tissue and are capable of reaching the lymph nodes under the arms. Once cancer has reached the lymph nodes, it has a route to go to other bodily regions.

Even though early-stage breast cancer often exhibits no symptoms, prompt discovery may transform a breast cancer narrative into one of survival.

Symptoms of breast Cancer include:
- A fresh bulge or lump in your breast, armpit, or collarbone area. However, certain lumps may be uncomfortable or sensitive. Most lumps are not painful. (Many lumps, however, are not breast cancer. Having your doctor check it is the only way to know.)
- Swollen breast.
- Irritation, dimpling, thickness, redness, or scaliness of the skin of your breast (which might make it resemble an orange peel).
- Discomfort in the breast or nipple.
- Non-breast milk nipple discharge.
- Nipple retraction (a "dented" or turned-inward nipple).

Not everyone who exhibits these symptoms has breast cancer. Therefore, if you observe any changes in your breasts, it's crucial to see your doctor or a breast expert.

Breast self-examination

You may learn how your breasts typically feel and appear by doing routine self-checks, which can help you spot changes as soon as they occur. Observe the following:

your breasts' overall size, shape, or color may vary.

skin that is dimpling or expanding, rash, or swelling, nipple inversion, or unusual discharge

Breast cancer types

The nature of breast cancer may be divided into two categories:

Cancer that has not spread from the source tissue is referred to as **noninvasive (in situ)** cancer. Stage 0 is used to describe this.

- Cancer that has spread to neighboring tissues is referred to as **invasive (infiltrating) cancer.** Based on how far it has spread, they are divided into stages 1, 2, 3, or 4.
- The kind of cancer is determined by the afflicted tissue. For instance:

- Ductal cancer. Cancer that develops in the milk ducts' lining is called **ductal carcinoma**. The most common kind of breast cancer is this one.
- lobular cancer Breast lobules may develop cancer, which is known as **lobular carcinoma**. Milk is made in the lobules.
- **Sarcoma**. This particular kind of cancer develops in the breast's connective tissue.
- **Angiosarcoma**. This kind begins in lymphatic or blood vessel lining cells.

Even if early symptoms and indicators are similar, breast cancer may also be divided into categories based on specific characteristics. Some of them are:

- Hormone-positive breast cancer. Estrogen and/or progesterone are the fuel for hormone-positive breast tumors.

- Breast cancer that is HER2-positive. A naturally occurring protein called the human epidermal growth factor promotes the proliferation of breast cancer cells. Your cancer is referred to as HER2-positive if it contains high amounts of this protein.

- Triple-negative breast cancer. Tests for HER2 and the estrogen, progesterone, and receptors are negative in triple-negative breast cancer.

- Breast cancer with papillary. Tiny papules finger-like growths are visible when papillary breast cancer is examined under a microscope. It might consist of cells that are both invasive and noninvasive.

- Breast metaplastic cancer. Along with aberrant ductal cells, metaplastic breast cancer may also include uncommon cell types including skin or bone cells. Usually, it is triple-negative.

Other than a breast lump, several kinds of breast cancer are more likely to exhibit symptoms. For instance:

- inflammatory breast cancer. Cancerous cells in breast skin restrict lymphatic arteries in inflammatory breast cancer. Its bloated, flaming, and inflamed appearance gives rise to its name.

- The breast illness Paget's The skin of the areola and nipple develops Paget's disease surrounding them. The region could seem scaly, crusty, or red. There might be a bloody or yellow discharge, and the nipple could flatten or invert. Burning or itching are some more signs.

- breast cancer that has spread. Breast cancer that has spread to distant areas of the body is referred to as metastatic breast cancer. The term "advanced" or "stage 4" breast cancer is also used. Loss of weight, unexplained discomfort, and weariness are some of the symptoms.

Breast Cancer In Men

Breast cancer is not often linked to those who were born with masculine gender identity. However, while it's more prevalent in older men, male breast cancer may happen in rare circumstances at any age.

Many individuals are unaware that everyone has breast cells and that those cells are capable of developing cancer. Breast cancer is less prevalent in this group of people because male breast cells are substantially less developed than female breast cells.

A lump in the breast tissue is the most typical indicator of breast cancer in persons who were given the gender of a man at birth. Male breast cancer symptoms include, in addition to a lump, thickening of the breast tissue, nipple discharge, and redness or scaling of the nipple.
Unexpected redness, swelling, skin irritation, itching, or a rash on the breast, as well as retracted or inward-turning nipples and enlarged lymph nodes under the arm

Male breast cancer is often discovered at a later stage because men may not routinely inspect their breast tissue for indicators of lumps.

Breast cancer treatment

Treatments might change depending on the kind and stage of cancer. But there are several standard methods that medical professionals and experts use to treat breast cancer:

1. When your doctor performs a lumpectomy, your breast is left unharmed.
2. A mastectomy is a surgical procedure in which your doctor removes all of the breast tissue, including the tumor and any attached tissue.
3. The most popular cancer treatment, chemotherapy, uses anticancer medications. These substances prevent cells from reproducing.
4. Radiation directly combats cancer by using radiation beams.
5. When HER2 or hormones are involved in the development of the malignancy,

hormone and targeted treatment may be employed.

2. Cancer of the brain

The proliferation of brain cells that causes brain tumors is known as brain cancer. Cancer, on the other hand, begins in another place of the body and progresses to the brain. It is referred to as secondary or metastasized brain cancer when that occurs.

Some malignant brain tumors have a rapid rate of growth. These cancerous tumors may interfere with how your body functions. Brain tumors should be treated as soon as they are discovered since they may be fatal.

Brain tumors are rather rare. People have a less than 1% lifetime risk of getting a malignant brain tumor, according to estimates from the American Cancer Society.

Symptoms of brain Cancer

The size and location of the brain tumor affect the symptoms of brain cancer. Particularly in its early stages, brain cancer exhibits many of the same symptoms as several less dangerous diseases.

Numerous of these symptoms are quite typical and are not likely to be signs of brain cancer. However, it's a good idea to see a doctor if you've had any of these symptoms for more than a week, if they came on abruptly, if they don't go away with over-the-counter painkillers, or if any of them worry you.

1. Common signs of brain cancer include nausea, vomiting, and headaches, which are often greater in the morning.
2. miscommunication
3. a loss of equilibrium
4. difficulty walking forgetfulness
5. thinking and speaking difficulties
6. vision issues
7. character alters

8. inconsistent eye motions
9. jerks or twitching of the muscles, inexplicable fainting, or syncope, and sleepiness
10. tingling or numbness in the arms or legs
11. seizures

Early diagnosis significantly improves the prognosis for brain cancer. If you often suffer any of the aforementioned symptoms or suspect that your symptoms may be more serious, schedule an appointment with a doctor right away for a diagnosis.

Brain Cancer Causes And Risk Factors

It is unclear what specifically causes primary brain cancer. However, research has linked ionizing radiation exposure at high levels to a higher chance of developing brain cancer. The most frequent sources of ionizing radiation include radiation therapy treatments, regular medical imaging tests (CT scans, X-rays), and potential employment exposure.

Increased age and a family history of brain cancer are two additional risk factors that may be linked to getting brain cancer.

Long-term smoking exposure to pesticides, herbicides, and fertilizers, as well as lead, plastic, rubber, petroleum, and certain fabrics that may have been contaminated with the Epstein-Barr virus or may have caused mononucleosis, may all contribute to cancer.

Some forms of cancer are more likely to produce secondary brain cancer than others, which is the kind of brain cancer that develops when cancer travels from another region of your body to your brain.

The following cancers often metastasize, or spread, to the brain:
- lung disease
- mammary cancer
- renal cancer
- urethral cancer
- melanoma, a kind of skin cancer.

brain tumor types

Names for brain tumors are determined by their location inside the brain or upper spine. A grade is also assigned to tumors. How quickly a tumor is anticipated to develop is indicated by its grade. Grades range from one to four, with four being the fastest-growing grades and one being the slowest.

Glioma is one of the most prevalent kinds of brain tumors. About 3 out of 10 occurrences of brain cancer are gliomas, which are brain tumors that start in the glial cells.

Astrocytoma.
Glioblastomas, the kind of quickly-expanding brain tumor, are a subtype of astrocytomas.

Meningioma.
Meningioma tumors, the most prevalent kind of brain tumor in adults, develop in the tissue that surrounds your brain and spinal cord and are often benign and slow-growing.

Ganglioglioma.
Surgery is often used to treat the slow-growing tumors known as gangliogliomas that are present in glial and neuronal cells.

Craniopharyngiomas. Craniopharyngiomas are slow-growing tumors that develop between the pituitary gland and the brain. Because they often encroach on the optic nerves, they may impair eyesight.

Schwannomas.
Almost typically benign, schwannomas are slow-growing tumors that develop around the cranial nerves.

Medulloblastoma.
Children are more likely to develop medulloblastomas, which are rapidly developing tumors that develop on the nerve cells in the brain.

How Is Cancer Of The Brain Detected?

Your physician may carry out one of the following procedures to determine if you have symptoms of a brain tumor:

a brain biopsy, which is a surgical procedure in which a small amount of the tumor is removed for diagnostic testing and to determine whether your tumor is malignant. A neurological examination to determine whether a tumor is affecting your brain imaging tests, such as CT, MRI, and positron emission tomography (PET) scans, to locate the tumor a lumbar puncture, which is a procedure that collects a small sample of the fluid that surrounds your brain and spinal cord, for the check.

How Is Cancer Of The Brain Treated?

Brain cancer may be treated in several ways. Primary brain cancer will be treated differently from cancer that has spread to other organs.

The kind, size, and location of your brain tumor will determine whether you get one therapy or more. There will also be considerations for your age and overall health.

Surgery

The most popular form of therapy for brain tumors is brain surgery. The tumor may be completely, partly, or not at all removed depending on its position.

Chemotherapy.
These medications may reduce your tumor and kill brain cancer cells. Chemotherapy may be administered orally or intravenously.

Radiation Treatment
This procedure employs high-energy radiation, such as X-rays, to kill cancer cells and tumor tissue that cannot be surgically removed.

Combo Treatment.
Combination treatment refers to the simultaneous administration of chemotherapy and radiation therapy.

Biologic Medicines

These medications support, guide, or restore your body's natural tumor defenses. For instance, immunotherapy is a kind of biological medication that is often prescribed and increases your immune system's capacity to recognize and fight cancer.

Different Medicines.

To address symptoms and adverse effects brought on by your brain tumor and brain cancer therapies, your doctor may prescribe drugs.

Rehabilitation.

If your ability to speak, move or do other everyday tasks has been impacted by your disease or treatment, you may need to go to rehabilitation sessions. Physical therapy, occupational therapy, and other treatments are all a part of rehabilitation and may assist you in learning skills.

substitute treatments.
There isn't a lot of scientific evidence to back up adopting complementary medicines to treat brain cancer. However, some medical experts do advise taking measures like eating a balanced diet and taking vitamin and mineral supplements to make up for nutrients lost during cancer therapy. Before changing your diet, taking any supplements or herbs, or pursuing any other alternative therapy, see your doctor.

Prevention Of Brain Cancer?
Although there is no known method to prevent brain cancer, you may lower your risk by staying away from:
exposure to carcinogenic substances, smoking, and pesticides and insecticides
radiation exposure that is not required.

3. Vaginal Cancer
A very uncommon form of cancer that begins in the vagina is vaginal cancer. The National Cancer Institute (NCI) estimates that it causes about 2% of female genital cancers.

Varieties of vaginal cancer

Savage cell. This kind of cancer slowly spreads throughout the vaginal lining. According to the American Cancer Society, it is responsible for roughly 9 out of 10 cases of vaginal cancer (ACS).

Adenocarcinoma. It begins in the cells of the vaginal gland. It is the second most prevalent kind of vaginal cancer and most frequently affects women over 50.

Melanoma. This kind of cancer begins in the cells that give skin color, just like the more prevalent melanoma skin cancer type.

Sarcoma. This only accounts for a small portion of vaginal cancers and begins in the vaginal walls.

Early vaginal cancer treatment has a high rate of success.

You'll notice that the terminology used to share statistics and other data is largely binary, alternating between the terms "female" and "women."

Although we generally try to avoid using language like this, being specific is important when discussing research participants and clinical outcomes.

Unfortunately, the research and polls cited in this book did not collect data from or include transgender, nonbinary, genderqueer, gender nonconforming, agender, or genderless individuals.

Vaginal Cancer Symptoms
However, cancer that has spread to other tissues usually manifests as symptoms.
The most typical type is unusual vaginal bleeding.
This includes bleeding after:
- Menopause.
- Bleeding during or after sex and occurs between periods.

- Also possible are heavier or longer-lasting bleeding.

Other signs comprise:
- Painful or frequent urination with blood- or odor-filled or watery vaginal discharge.
- pelvic discomfort, particularly with sexual activity.
- A lump or mass in the vagina.
- Persistent vaginal itching.
- Constipation.
- Back discomfort stool or pee containing blood.
- Leg swelling.
- Fistulas in advanced stage cancer.

It's important to see a doctor or other healthcare professional (HCP) to rule out potential causes of many of these symptoms as cancer isn't the only possibility.

Who is susceptible to vaginal cancer? What causes it?

In most instances, according to the ACS, the precise etiology is unclear.

But the following has been connected to vaginal cancer:

HIV (human papillomavirus) (HPV): The National Health Service states that this STD is the primary sexually transmitted disease responsible for vaginal cancer. According to Cancer Research UK, HPV is safe for the majority of individuals. But over time, chronic infection with high-risk virus strains may lead to cancer.

A history of cervical cancer: Also often linked to cervical cancer is HPV.

Diethylstilbestrol exposure during pregnancy (DES): This drug used to be administered to expectant mothers to lower the risk of miscarriage. But in the 1970s, medical professionals ceased recommending it. Nowadays, DES-related vaginal cancer is quite uncommon.

There are other risk factors for vaginal cancer, such as:

- A weakened immune system, which can be brought on by diseases like HIV or lupus early exposure to HPV through sexual activity.
- Changes in the cells that line the vagina.
- Having had a previous hysterectomy, whether it was for a benign or malignant mass.
- Smoking, which the ACS says more than doubles the risk of vaginal cancer.
- Age — it's rare in people younger than 40.

Even if you have one of these risk factors, you may not have vaginal cancer. Similarly, even if you don't have any of them, vaginal cancer still has a chance to strike.

Staging

The stages of vaginal cancer indicate how far the disease has progressed. In addition to the precancerous stage, there are four primary phases of vaginal cancer:

Neoplasia of the vaginal intraepithelium (VAIN). Precancers include VAIN. Although there are aberrant cells in the vaginal lining, they have not yet begun to proliferate or spread. Not cancer, VAIN.

Stage 1. Only the vaginal wall is prone to cancer.

Stage 2. Cancer has reached nearby tissue but has not yet reached the pelvic wall.

Stage 3. Cancer has penetrated the pelvic wall and more of the pelvis. Additionally, adjacent lymph nodes may have been affected.

Stage 4:

There are two phases within Cancer that are at stage 4.

Stage 4A has progressed to the bladder, the rectum, or both.

In stage 4B, cancer has progressed to distant lymph nodes, the liver, the lungs, and other organs.

In What Ways Is Vaginal Cancer Treated?
Surgery to remove the tumor and a little portion of good tissue surrounding it may be necessary if

the cancer is stage 1 and located in the upper part of the vagina. Radiotherapy is often administered next.

In all stages of vaginal cancer, radiotherapy is the most often prescribed therapy. In rare circumstances, chemotherapy may be given in addition to radiation. Chemotherapy for vaginal cancer, however, is not well supported by research.

A doctor or other HCP will probably advise surgery if you've previously had radiation in the vaginal region. This is so that each component of the body only experiences a limited quantity of radiation.

Although stage 4b cancer is often incurable, therapy may reduce symptoms. In this situation, a physician or other HCP may advise radiation or chemotherapy.

Radiotherapy

You may feel the following during treatment and for a short period after it ends, according to

Cancer Research UK, since radiation may harm both healthy and malignant cells:

- Fatigue.
- Discomfort in the region being treated.
- Pain while urinating.
- diarrhea and/or vomiting
- vaginal discharge

Radiotherapy may also have an impact on your sexual life because it can produce scar tissue, which can make intercourse painful by making the vagina smaller.

Further pain during intercourse might result from vaginal dryness.

In this regard, your medical staff ought to be able to assist you by providing things like lubricants and dilators.

Your bladder's elasticity might also deteriorate. Your need to urinate can increase.

Additionally, external radiation to the pelvis might hasten the onset of menopause, preventing you from becoming pregnant. Early menopausal women may still have children via adoption and surrogacy, among other options.

Surgery

All types of surgery have the potential for postoperative discomfort as well as an increased risk of infection and blood clots. However, smaller operations often carry fewer hazards than larger ones.

Sexuality may be impacted.

The vaginal lining won't be able to generate mucus if you get a vaginal reconstruction. To prevent dryness and irritation during sexual activity, you'll probably need to apply lubricant.

Scar tissue may also make the vaginal opening smaller. Penetrative vaginal intercourse may become more painful and challenging as a result.

The bladder or rectum may need to be removed in specific circumstances. You'll need to eliminate your waste with a different approach if this occurs. Your stomach may be cut open by a surgeon, who will then put a colostomy bag on it to collect waste.

The rectum may sometimes be rebuilt, making a colostomy bag merely a temporary solution.

Additional dangers associated with surgical therapy include:

- If your groin lymph nodes are removed, you're more likely to have lymphedema or swollen legs.
- You're also more likely to experience early menopause if your ovaries are removed.

Chemotherapy

Radiotherapy and chemotherapy both have a similar set of adverse effects. It may also harm healthy cells.

Some adverse consequences are:

- Dizziness or vomiting.
- Tiredness.
- Breathlessness.
- Greater risk of infections with thinning or lost hair.

Getting rid of ovarian cancer?

There are things you may do to help minimize your risk of vaginal cancer even if you might not be able to eliminate it:

Take action to reduce your HPV risk. This includes receiving the HPV vaccination and using condoms and other barrier techniques anytime you engage in any form of sexual activity (vaginal, oral, or anal).

If you smoke, you may want to stop. Smoking is a significant lifestyle risk factor for malignancies, including vaginal cancer. Here are some pointers to get you going.

- Only drink in moderation. Heavy drinking may raise your risk of vaginal cancer, according to some research.

- Get frequent Pap tests and pelvic examinations. This will assist your doctor or another HCP in identifying precancers before they develop into vaginal malignancies or early detection of vaginal cancer before spread or the emergence of troubling symptoms.

4. Cancer Of The lungs.

The second most frequent malignancy among Americans is lung cancer. In addition, it is the main reason for cancer-related fatalities in both men and women in the US.

Lung cancer causes 1 in 4 cancer-related fatalities, according to the American Lung Association.

Lung cancer is mostly brought on by cigarette smoking. Lung cancer is 23 times more likely to strike men who smoke than nonsmokers. Women are 13 times more likely to smoke.

Because of improved early diagnosis and individuals stopping smoking, the number of new lung cancer cases is declining in the United States.

Lung cancer symptoms include:
1. A cough that won't go away and keeps getting worse over time.
2. Exhaling blood.

3. Breathing difficulties or wheezing.
4. Chronic chest pain
5. bone ache.
6. Vocal changes such as hoarseness.
7. Consistent lung infections (like pneumonia or bronchitis).
8. Shedding pounds without trying.
9. I'M not hungry.
10. Chronic headaches.
11. Clots of blood.

Typically, lung cancer doesn't present symptoms until it has progressed (also referred to as late-stage cancer). That's because tumors may develop in your lungs without making you feel any discomfort since they have few nerve endings. Consult your doctor if you have any of the aforementioned symptoms so they can check you for lung cancer and other potential causes, such as asthma.

Lung Cancer Types
Lung cancer comes in various distinct forms. Small-cell lung cancer (SCLC) or non-small cell lung cancer (NSCLC) make up the majority of

lung cancer subtypes (SCLC). However, both types of cells may be seen in some people's malignancies.

1. Non-small cell lung cancer (NSCLC): Between 80 and 85 percent of cases are NSCLC. NSCLC comes in a variety of forms. If detected in the early stages, the majority of NSCL types respond well to therapy.

2. About 30% of all instances of non-small cell lung cancer (NSCLC) start in the cells that line the respiratory system passageways. Squamous cell lung carcinoma. Squamous cell carcinoma is the term for this.

3. Adenocarcinomas: These often develop in the lungs' outermost layer.

4. Adenocarcinoma in situ (AIS) is a rare kind of adenocarcinoma that starts in the lungs' tiny air sacs. It isn't aggressive and

may not need emergency medical attention.

5. Adenosquamous carcinoma: This malignancy appears in squamous cells and cells that secrete mucus.

6. Large cell carcinomas are a rapidly expanding subset of NSCLCs that fall beyond the scope of other cancer types.

7. About 15 to 20 percent of lung tumors are small-cell lung cancers (SCLC). Compared to NSCLC, this kind of lung cancer is more aggressive. Even while SCLC often responds to treatment more favorably at first, it is less likely to be cured than NSCLC.

8. Mesothelioma: Asbestos exposure is a risk factor for developing this kind of lung cancer. It happens when hormone-producing (neuroendocrine) cells give rise to carcinoid tumors.

Mesothelioma spreads quickly and with aggression. Treatment has not been successful in curing it.

lung cancer stages.

When lung cancer is detected and treated early, the likelihood of successful or curative therapy is significantly increased. The diagnosis of lung cancer often occurs after it has progressed since it may not present with clear symptoms in the early stages.

Stages of non-small cell lung cancer (NSCLC)

Cancer is discovered in the lung at stage 1, but it has not gone elsewhere.

Stage 2: Lymph nodes close by and the lung has cancer.

Stage 3: Lymph nodes in the center of the chest and a lung are both affected by cancer.

Stage 3A: Only on the side of the chest where cancer originally began to spread are lymph nodes discovered to be cancerous.

Stage 3B: Cancer has progressed to the lymph nodes above the collarbone or on the other side of the chest.

Cancer has progressed to both lungs, the region around the lungs, or distant organs at stage 4.

Stages of small-cell lung cancer (SCLC):
The SCLC process has two stages: limited and extended. Cancer is only discovered in one lung or close-by lymph nodes on the same side of the chest at the restricted stage.

When cancer is at the widespread stage, it has progressed across one lung, to the opposing lung, to the opposing side's lymph nodes, to the fluid surrounding the lung, to the bone marrow, and distant organs.

The widespread stage of SCLC is present in around 2 out of 3 patients at the time of diagnosis.

How Cancer of the lung is treated
Surgery to remove the tumor and chemotherapy and radiation therapy to eradicate cancer cells

are the main lung cancer therapies. Modern cancer therapies including targeted therapy and immunotherapy are sometimes employed, but often only at advanced stages.

Non-small cell lung cancer (NSCLC) therapy generally differs from patient to patient. The specifics of your health and the stage of your cancer at the time of diagnosis will determine your treatment approach.

According to the stage, NSCLC treatment options often include:

- Stage 1 NSCLC: You may just need surgery to remove a piece of the lung. Additionally, chemotherapy can be suggested, particularly if your risk of recurrence is high. If discovered at this time, cancer is most easily treated.

- Stage 2 NSCLC: Your lung may need to be partially or completely removed after surgery. Usually, chemotherapy is advised.

- You could need a combination of chemotherapy, surgery, and radiation therapy for stage 3 NSCLC.

- Surgery, radiation, chemotherapy, targeted treatment, and immunotherapy is available for stage 4 NSCLC.

Surgery, chemotherapy, and radiation therapy are other treatment options for small-cell lung cancer (SCLC). The malignancy will often be too advanced for surgery in most situations.

If you are given a lung cancer diagnosis, your care will probably be overseen by a group of medical professionals that may include:

1. An expert surgeon in the chest and lungs (thoracic surgeon).
2. A lung professional (pulmonologist).
3. An oncologist in medicine.
4. A radio oncologist.

Before choosing a course of therapy, discuss all of your alternatives. Your physicians will communicate with one another and coordinate treatment.

Home remedies for symptoms of lung cancer
Cancer cannot be cured by home treatments. Some, however, could be able to ease lung cancer symptoms or adverse effects from therapy. Alternatives include:

1. Massage: A massage may help reduce stress and discomfort. Some massage therapists have received special training to assist cancer patients.

2. Acupuncture: When carried out by a skilled professional, acupuncture may improve discomfort and reduce nausea and vomiting. If you use blood thinners or have low blood counts, it's not safe.

3. Reflection and relaxation may lower stress and enhance the general quality of life.

4. Yoga: By including breathing exercises, meditation, and stretching, yoga may enhance your mood and sleep.

5. Cannabis oil: According to some, using cannabis oil helps with hunger, nausea relief, and pain management. However, these assertions need more study. This choice isn't accessible everywhere since different states have different marijuana regulations.

6. Dietary advice for those with lung cancer

7. No diet can reduce the risk of lung cancer. Nevertheless, it's crucial to consume all the nutrients your body requires.

You may have appetite loss as a result of cancer therapies. They may also hinder your body's ability to absorb vitamins. If you're lacking in a certain vitamin, your doctor may suggest specific meals or supplements for you.

Here are some nutritional suggestions:

- Eat anytime you are hungry.
- Try eating smaller meals throughout the day if you don't feel hungry.
- Supplement with low-sugar, high-calorie meals and beverages if you need to put on weight.
- Teas with mint and ginger might help to settle your stomach.
- Avoid spicy meals if you have mouth sores or a sensitive stomach.
- Increase your intake of high-fiber meals if constipation is a concern.

Your tolerance to certain foods may fluctuate as your therapy progresses. Likewise, your side effects and dietary requirements. It's important to talk to your doctor about nutrition. You may also request a recommendation for a dietitian or nutritionist.

5. Prostate Cancer

The most frequent kind of cancer among men is prostate cancer. In the US, the American Cancer Society (ACS) predicts that in 2022, there will be 268,490 new cases of this illness in males.

The prostate is a little gland that may be found in the lower abdomen of males, next to the bladder and urethra. The prostate is regulated by the hormone testosterone. In addition, the prostate gland produces semen or seminal fluid. When a man ejaculates, semen, which contains sperm, leaves the urethra.

Prostate cancer occurs when a tumor, or abnormal, malignant development of cells, develops in the prostate. Other parts of the body may get infected with this malignancy. In these situations, the cancer is nevertheless referred to be prostate cancer since it is comprised of cells from the prostate.

Symptoms of prostate cancer
1. Problems peeing, such as difficulty beginning or holding back urination, leakage, interrupted urine flow, or a sudden, irresistible need to urinate are examples of warning signs.
2. Urination-related discomfort, which may seem like a burning feeling.

3. Frequent urination, particularly during the night.
4. Difficulty attaining or maintaining an erection.
5. Alterations in ejaculation, such as discomfort or a decrease in the volume of fluid ejected.
6. Pee or ejaculate with blood in it.
7. Your lower back, thighs, hips, or pelvic region may be painful.
8. Rectal pressure or discomfort.

Typically, there aren't any early warning indications of prostate cancer. If you are a guy over the age of 55 and have no symptoms, experts advise that you speak to your doctor about being tested for the condition. Visit your doctor straight away if you have any symptoms. These signs may also be brought on by other conditions like prostatitis (inflammation of the prostate).

Prostate Cancer Types

Adenocarcinoma, a kind of cancer that develops in the tissue of a gland like the prostate gland, accounts for the majority of occurrences of prostate cancer. However, the prostate may also be the site of several uncommon cancers, such as:

- such as lung cancer, small cell carcinoma
- Sarcomas, such as bone cell cancer.
- Transitional cell carcinomas, such as pancreatic cancer.
- Neuroendocrine tumors

The rate of growth of prostate cancer is another classification. It grows in two ways: aggressively, or quickly, and nonaggressively, or slowly.

The tumor grows gradually in nonaggressive prostate cancer. Aggressive cancer, on the other hand, may cause the tumor to overgrow, spread to other parts of the body like the bones, and develop into metastatic cancer.

Causes and risk factors for prostate cancer
Although there is no known cause of prostate cancer, risk factors including age or family

history may make you more likely to have the disease.

Who is in danger?

Although any man might get prostate cancer, there are specific variables that increase your risk. These risk elements consist of:

Older age, 50 or older, a family history of prostate cancer, certain ethnic or racial groups (for example, African American guys are more likely to develop prostate cancer due to obesity genetic alterations), and

Some studies take into account other risk variables including nutrition and chemical exposure that may raise your likelihood of being diagnosed. The ACS claims that these impacts are currently unknown. Additionally uncommon among males under the age of 40 is prostate cancer.

Stages Of Prostate cancer

Using a staging method, your doctor may describe how far cancer has spread.

Prostate cancer is staged using the American Joint Committee on Cancer (AJCC) TMN staging approach. The system stages it by, like many other cancer types:

- The tumor's size or degree of lymph node involvement.
- Regardless of whether cancer has spread (metastasized) to other locations or organs.
- Around the time of diagnosis, the PSA level.
- Gleason rating.

There are 1 to 4 stages of prostate cancer. However, stage 4 is when the illness is most advanced.

Treatments For Prostate Cancer

Based on your age, health, and the stage of your cancer, your doctor will create a suitable treatment plan for you.

Nonaggressive

Your doctor could advise active monitoring, often known as watchful waiting if the cancer is non-aggressive. This means you'll postpone treatment while continuing to monitor your cancer with frequent medical visits.

Every six months, your doctor will assess your PSA and do an annual DRE if they decide to monitor your cancer using active surveillance. In addition, one to three years after the original diagnosis, they could do another biopsy and imaging.

When just watching the condition, the doctor actively observes your symptoms to determine if therapy is necessary.

Aggressive

Other methods, such as surgery, are sometimes used by doctors to treat more severe forms of cancer. Such as:

- Radiation
- Hormone treatment with cryotherapy
- Chemotherapy
- Staging-based radiosurgery
- Immunotherapy

Your bones may have been affected by bone metastasis if your cancer is very aggressive and has spread. The aforementioned therapies, along with others, may be used for bone metastases.

Prostatectomy

A prostatectomy is a surgical treatment when your prostate gland is partially or completely removed. For instance, your doctor could advise a radical prostatectomy, which involves removing the whole prostate, if you have prostate cancer that hasn't progressed outside of the prostate.

Different radical prostatectomies are available. Some are open, so your lower abdomen will be covered by a longer incision. Others are laparoscopic, so your stomach will be cut in many tiny places.

Prostate Cancer prevention

You have no control over certain prostate cancer risk factors, including age and family history. Others, however, you could handle.

For instance, giving up smoking may lower your chance of developing prostate cancer. Exercise and proper diet are other important elements that might affect your chances of developing prostate cancer.

Diet

A diet low in dairy and calcium is one item that may help lower your risk of prostate cancer. You may reduce your risk of prostate cancer by eating certain foods, such as:
fish that is made with cruciferous vegetables like kale, broccoli, and Brussels sprouts, omega-3 fatty acid-rich soy oils, such as olive oil

Exercise

Your chance of acquiring advanced prostate cancer and passing away from prostate cancer may probably be lowered with exercise.
Exercise may also aid in weight loss, which is important given that obesity has been linked to a higher risk of prostate cancer according to studies from 2016. Aim for 30 minutes of

exercise on most days of the week with your doctor's consent.

Consult your physician.

All men are at risk for prostate cancer as they get older, but the prognosis is often excellent if it is detected and treated early. Therefore, as you age, be important, to be frank with your doctor about your risk.

Consult your doctor straight away if you have any symptoms you believe might be related to prostate cancer. Additionally, even if you are symptom-free, think about changing to a healthy lifestyle to lower your risk.

6. Colon Cancer

Cancerous cells in the rectum may evolve into rectal cancer. The rectum is situated above the anus and under the sigmoid colon.

The digestive system includes both your rectum and colon, hence tumors of both are sometimes referred to as colorectal cancers.

Colorectal cancer is the third most prevalent cancer in the country. Considering that it's also the second-deadliest, early identification and treatment are essential. According to statistics from the Worldwide Cancer Research Fund from 2020, the colorectal disease is the second most frequent cancer in women worldwide and the third most common cancer in men.

In the United States, there are expected to be 44,850 new cases of rectal cancer in 2022, according to the American Cancer Society. 106,180 new instances of colon cancer are comparable to this.

What are the signs and symptoms of colorectal Cancer?

Rectal cancer may initially show no symptoms. Rectal bleeding is the most typical symptom when the malignancy becomes worse. Your bowel habits might change and stay that way for a while. Additionally, you can feel unjustified weariness and weakness.

The Centers for Disease Control and Prevention (CDC) list the following as typical signs of colorectal cancer:

- Rectal bleeding variations in how often you urinate sensation like your bowels aren't emptying fully discomfort when you urinate
- constipation or diarrhea
- stool that contains blood or mucus, unexpected appetite changes, and weight loss
- inexplicable exhaustion, frequent gas, cramps, and pain in the abdomen
- Iron deficiency anemia, which may happen as a consequence of blood loss, is another indication that you may have rectal cancer.

What causes Rectal Cancer?

Malignant tumors form when cancerous cells proliferate and expand out of control, while the precise etiology of rectal cancer is uncertain. These cells can infiltrate and eliminate healthy tissue. Sometimes it's unclear what initiates this process.

Some inherited gene mutations may make you more likely to develop rectal cancer. **Hereditary nonpolyposis colorectal cancer** (HNPCC), sometimes referred to as Lynch syndrome, is one of them. The risk of colon and other cancers is considerably increased by this disease. Your doctor could advise colon removal as a preventative strategy in certain circumstances.

Familial Adenomatous Polyposis is another hereditary disorder that may result in rectal cancer (FAP). The lining of the colon and rectum may develop polyps as a result of this uncommon illness.

While initially benign, these polyps have the potential to develop into a malignancy. In actuality, the majority of FAP patients get cancer before the age of 50. A large bowel removal procedure can also be suggested by your doctor as a prophylactic measure.

The stages of rectal cancer are listed here.
Cancer is staged to show how far along it is, which might assist physicians in selecting the most effective course of action.

Stage 0 (carcinoma in situ)
Unusual cells are only present in the rectum wall's deepest layer.
Despite not reaching lymph nodes, **stage 1** cancer cells have penetrated the deepest layer of the rectum wall.

Stage 2
Although lymph nodes have not been affected, cancer cells have penetrated or entered the outer muscular layer of the rectum wall. This is often known as stage 2A. The malignancy has entered the abdominal lining at stage 2B.

Stage 3
One or more lymph nodes have had cancerous cells spread from the rectum's outermost muscle layer. Depending on how much lymph node

tissue is impacted, stage 3 is sometimes divided into substages 3A, 3B, and 3C.

Cancer cells in **stage 4** have migrated to distant organs like the liver or lungs.

What are the stages of therapy available?

The doctor and the rest of the care team will take into account: your age, the extent of any possible malignancy, and your overall health

The time of each therapy as well as the ideal treatment combination may be decided upon using this information.

Treatment for Rectal Cancer

The general recommendations for therapy are shown below per stage. There are possible treatments on this list. The therapy choices that are given for each stage may not be necessary for all patients.

Stage 0

1. Colonoscopy removal of questionable tissue.

2. Tissue removal during a different operation
3. Tissue and a portion of the surrounding region are removed

Stage 1
For certain individuals, local excision or resection radiation treatment some individuals get chemotherapy.

Stages 2 and 3.
Surgery, radiation treatment, and chemotherapy in stages 2 and 3.

Stage 4
- surgery and radiation treatment, maybe in more than one part of the body
- chemotherapy targeted treatments, such as angiogenesis inhibitors or monoclonal antibodies.
- Cryosurgery, in which defective tissue is destroyed using a cold liquid or a cryoprobe, and radiofrequency ablation, in

which unwanted cells are eliminated using radio waves
- palliative care to enhance the overall quality of life, such as a stent to maintain the rectum open if a tumor blocks it

What can be done to avoid rectal cancer?
Your chances of survival might be increased if you get a colon cancer diagnosis in its early stages before it spreads.

The American Cancer Society and the Centers for Disease Control and Prevention (CDC) advise starting routine screenings at age 45 to significantly lower your overall risk of acquiring colorectal cancer. Your doctor could advise testing earlier than this, based on your family history, genetics, and other risk factors.

When detected via standard screenings, such as a normal colonoscopy or stool test, colon and rectal cancer may be caught early. Very sensitive stool tests may find cancer. A timely colonoscopy should also be done if abnormal cells are found.

By leading a healthy lifestyle and avoiding risk factors including inactivity, smoking, and consuming red or processed meats, you may also be able to prevent rectal cancer.

7. Gastric Cancer

When malignant cells proliferate inside the stomach lining, stomach cancer develops. This form of cancer, also known as gastric cancer, may be difficult to identify since the majority of patients seldom exhibit symptoms in the early stages. As a consequence, it often remains undetected until it has spread to other bodily areas.

The National Cancer Institute (NCI) estimates that 27,000 new cases of stomach cancer will be diagnosed in 2021. Additionally, the NCI calculated that 1.4% of all new cancer cases in the US were stomach cancer.

It's crucial to get the information you need to manage the condition even though stomach cancer may be challenging to identify and cure.

Why Does Stomach Cancer Develop?

One portion of the upper digestive system is made up of your stomach and esophagus. The task of digesting food and transferring the nutrients to the other parts of your digestive system, notably the small and large intestines, is carried out by your stomach.

When healthy cells in the upper digestive tract become malignant and proliferate out of control, developing a tumor, stomach cancer develops. Typically, this procedure proceeds slowly. Stomach cancer often takes years to grow.

Signs Of Gastric Cancer

The American Cancer Society states that stomach cancer often has no early indications or symptoms. As a result, individuals often don't notice anything is wrong until the disease has progressed.

There could be illness signs in various situations. The following are some of the most typical signs of stomach cancer:

- chronic heartburn
- reduced appetite
- early satiety, frequent burping, and persistent bloating (feeling full after eating only a small amount)
- extreme tiredness
- chronic stomach ache

Many of these symptoms are typical of other illnesses, such as an infection or an ulcer. As a result, diagnosing stomach cancer may be challenging. It's crucial to contact a doctor if you have stomach cancer symptoms that may not improve.

Stomach Cancer Stages

The stomach cancer stage reveals the extent of the disease's internal dissemination.

The American Joint Committee on Cancer's TNM staging approach is often used to assess the stage of stomach cancer. The system examines three things:

T category: the tumor's dimensions and extent

N category: the extent of the lymph node cancer spread

Whether cancer has spread to distant parts of the body falls under the M category.

Each category's results are combined to assign a stage from 0 to 4. An earlier stage of cancer is indicated by a lower number. Although tumor development and spread will vary, each stage generally resembles:

Stage 0. Only the surface of the stomach lining has abnormal or malignant cells, and the disease has not migrated to the lymph nodes or other organs.

Stage 1: The tumor has grown into the stomach's deeper layers. The lymph nodes around the stomach may or may not have picked up cancer, but it hasn't migrated to any other organs.

Stage 2. Cancer has often progressed to the lymph nodes and the tumor has penetrated deeper layers of the stomach. It hasn't expanded to other bodily regions.

Stage 3: The tumor has penetrated farther into the stomach's layers and may have spread to neighboring organs. Although it hasn't yet migrated to distant areas of the body, cancer has probably progressed to the lymph nodes.

Stage 4. The disease may have spread to surrounding or deeper stomach layers, although this is not necessary. At this point, cancer has migrated to distant organs such as the liver, brain, or lungs.

Cancer will be at a stage 0 to 3 if it hasn't spread to other places of the body. Stage 4 stomach cancer will be the prognosis if it has progressed to other regions.
Treatments and predicted survival rates vary according to the stage. 5 years after diagnosis, there is a 69.9% chance of surviving with early-stage cancer that is limited to the stomach. The 5-year likelihood of survival for cancer at a later stage that has spread to distant parts of the body lowers to 5.5%.

Gastric Cancer Treatment

Treatment for stomach cancer often includes one or more of the following:

Immunotherapy, which boosts or increases your immune system's capacity to fight cancer, includes chemotherapy, radiation therapy, surgery, and other treatments.

The kind and stage of your cancer will determine your precise treatment strategy. Age and general health might also be important factors.

The aim of therapy, in addition to treating stomach cancer cells, is to stop the cells from spreading. If stomach cancer is not treated, it may progress to: bones, liver, lymph nodes, and lungs

Prevention Of Stomach Cancer

There is no one way to avoid stomach cancer. Nevertheless, you may lessen your chance of getting any kind of cancer by:
- keeping a healthy weight.
- Eating a balanced diet.
- Using alcohol in moderation.

- Quitting smoking and exercising consistently.

In certain circumstances, physicians may recommend drugs that might aid in reducing the risk of stomach cancer. People who have precancerous conditions or other disorders that also benefit from the drug often undergo this.

An early screening test can also be something you want to think about. This examination may be useful in detecting stomach cancer.

One of the stomach cancer screening tests listed below may be used by a clinician to look for symptoms of the condition:

- Lab examinations for the body, such as blood and urine testing.
- X-rays and endoscopies, in which a tube with a lens is inserted down your throat to examine for any abnormalities, are examples of imaging procedures.
- Genetic analysis.

8. Bladder Cancer

The tissues of the bladder, the part of the body that stores pee, are where bladder cancer develops. Each year, the condition affects around 45,000 men and 17,000 women, according to the National Institutes of Health.

Symptoms include:

- Pee with blood in it. Typically, this is the initial indication of bladder cancer. Urine containing blood may appear pink, crimson, or orange.

- Alterations in urination, such as difficulty urinating, a weak urine stream, discomfort when peeing, or the inability to urinate.

If you have any of these issues, see your doctor. A urinary tract infection, an overactive bladder, or an enlarged prostate are a few more potential factors to be aware of.

Bladder Cancer Types

Bladder cancer may be one of three types:

Tumor with transitional cells

Among bladder cancers, transitional cell carcinoma is the most prevalent. It starts in the transitional cells that make up the bladder's inner layer. When tissue is stretched, cells are called transitional cells to shift form without becoming harmed.

Cancer Of The Squamous Cell

In the US, squamous cell carcinoma is an uncommon kind of cancer. After a protracted infection or bladder irritation, it starts when thin, flat squamous cells grow in the bladder.

Adenocarcinoma

Another uncommon cancer in the US is adenocarcinoma. It starts when glandular cells develop in the bladder during protracted bladder inflammation and irritation. The mucus-secreting glands in the body are made of glandular cells.

Stages of bladder Cancer

To determine how far the disease has gone, your doctor may stage your bladder cancer using a scale that ranges from stage 0 to stage 4. The following are the bladder cancer stages:

Bladder cancer that is at stage 0 has not progressed beyond the bladder's lining.
- Stage 1 bladder cancer has progressed through the bladder's lining but hasn't yet gotten to the muscular layer.
- The bladder's layer of muscle has been affected by stage 2 bladder cancer.
- The bladder's surrounding tissues have been affected by stage 3 bladder cancer.
- Stage 4 bladder cancer has progressed outside of the bladder to other body parts.

How is bladder cancer treated?
Based on the kind and stage of your bladder cancer, your symptoms, and your general health, your doctor will work with you to determine what therapy to provide.

Stage 0 And Stage 1 Treatment

Surgery to remove the bladder tumor is one kind of treatment for bladder cancer in stages 0 and 1, along with chemotherapy and immunotherapy, which includes taking a drug that triggers your immune system to fight the cancer cells.

Stage 2 And Stage 3 Treatment

In addition to chemotherapy, stage 2 and stage 3 bladder cancer patients may also have partial bladder removal.

Radiation therapy, chemotherapy, or immunotherapy can be used to shrink the tumor before surgery, treat cancer when surgery is not an option, kill any cancer cells that remain after surgery, or prevent cancer from returning.

Removal of the entire bladder, which is known as a radical cystectomy, followed by surgery to create a new way for urine to exit the body.

Stage 4 bladder cancer treatment.

Radiation therapy, immunotherapy, and chemotherapy may be used after surgery to kill any remaining cancer cells or to relieve symptoms and prolong life in stage 4 bladder cancer patients with radical cystectomy and removal of the surrounding lymph nodes, followed by surgery to create a new way for urine to exit the body.

Prevention of bladder cancer
Bladder cancer may not always be avoidable since physicians don't yet know what causes it. Your chance of developing bladder cancer may be decreased by the following elements and habits:
- not a smoker
- avoiding smoke from other cigarettes
- avoiding more cancer-causing substances
- consuming a lot of water

9. Liver cancer
Cancer that develops in the liver is known as liver cancer. Your biggest internal organ is the liver. It carries out some vital tasks that support your body's ability to digest food, absorb nutrients, and repair injuries.

Under your ribs in the upper right corner of your belly is where the liver is situated. It is in charge of creating bile, a fluid that aids in the digestion of fats, vitamins, and other nutrients.

Additionally, this important organ stores nutrients like glucose so that you may still be fed even when you aren't eating. Additionally, it decomposes poisons and drugs.

When liver cancer takes hold, it kills liver cells and impairs the liver's capacity to function normally.

Generally speaking, liver cancer is categorized as primary or secondary. In the liver's cells, primary liver cancer first appears. When cancer cells from another organ metastasize or move to the liver, secondary liver cancer occurs.

Cancer cells may separate from the main site, or where cancer first started, unlike other types of cells in your body.

The lymphatic system or bloodstream are two ways that the cells might move to different parts of your body. They may start to proliferate in other organs or tissues once they get there.

Liver Cancer Types

Primary liver cancer comes in a variety of forms. Each one is associated with a particular area of the liver or a particular kind of liver cell that is impacted. Primary liver cancer might begin as a single lump developing in your liver or it can begin simultaneously in several locations throughout your liver.

Primary liver carcinoma mostly manifests as:

Liver Cellular Cancer

The most typical form of liver cancer is hepatocellular carcinoma (HCC), sometimes referred to as hepatoma. The HCC type accounts for around 85 to 90 percent of primary liver malignancies. The primary cells that make up your liver, called hepatocytes, are where this problem originates.

People who have cirrhosis or long-term (chronic) hepatitis are substantially more prone to develop HCC. Hepatitis B or C infection is the most common factor that leads to cirrhosis, a devastating type of liver disease, heavy drinking for a long time and alcohol-unrelated fatty liver disease

Cholangiocarcinoma
The tiny, tube-like bile ducts in your liver are where cholangiocarcinoma, more generally referred to as bile duct cancer, originates. To aid in digestion, bile is transported via these ducts to the gallbladder.

It is known as intrahepatic bile duct carcinoma when cancer first appears in the portion of the ducts within your liver. Extrahepatic bile duct cancer refers to cancer that first appears in the portion of the ducts that are external to your liver.

Bile duct cancer is uncommon. About 8,000 Americans are given the diagnosis with it each year.

Liver Angiomatosis
A relatively uncommon kind of liver cancer called hepatic angiosarcoma starts in the blood veins of your liver. Due to the rapid progression

of this form of cancer, it is often discovered when it is more advanced.

Hepatoblastoma

Hepatoblastoma is a very uncommon kind of liver cancer. Nearly all children, particularly those under age 3, have it. Hepatoblastoma may be treated in around 70% of cases with surgery and chemotherapy.

What are the origins of liver cancer and its risk factors?

Why some individuals get liver cancer while others do not is a mystery to doctors. However, several elements have been linked to an increased risk of liver cancer, including:

- Age. Older persons are more likely to get liver cancer.
- Ethnicity and race. American Indians and Alaska Natives are more likely to get liver cancer than other ethnic groups in the country. In white individuals, it is the least prevalent.

- heavy drinking. Your chance of developing liver cancer rises with prolonged heavy drinking.
- Smoking. Your chance of developing liver cancer rises if you smoke cigarettes.
- exposure to aflatoxin A form of mold that may develop on wheat, maize, and peanuts can generate a poison called aflatoxin. Food handling regulations in the US restrict aflatoxin exposure on a large scale. In certain places, the exposure could be greater.
- usage of anabolic steroids. The risk of liver cancer rises with prolonged usage of anabolic steroids, a kind of synthetic testosterone.

Ailments Connected To Liver Cancer

Hepatitis: Hepatitis B or C infection that lasts a long time might seriously harm your liver.

Direct contact with the blood or semen of a person who has the virus may transmit hepatitis from one person to another.

It could also be transmitted during delivery from a giving parent to their fetus.

The use of condoms during sexual activity may reduce your chances of contracting hepatitis B and C.

Additionally, there is a vaccination that may save you against hepatitis B.

Cirrhosis: A kind of liver injury known as cirrhosis occurs when healthy tissue is replaced by damaged tissue.

An impaired liver's ability to function may eventually result in consequences like liver cancer.

The two most frequent causes of cirrhosis in the US are chronic, severe alcohol consumption and hepatitis C.

In the US, cirrhosis is a common precursor to liver cancer in the majority of cases.

diabetes type 2: When additional risk factors are present, type 2 diabetes may raise the chance of liver cancer.

diseases associated with obesity. Metabolic syndrome and non-alcoholic fatty liver disease, both of which increase the risk of liver cancer, are linked to obesity.

Genetic Disorders: The risk of liver cancer is increased by a variety of uncommon hereditary disorders, including:

- Illnesses associated with inadequate alpha-1.
- Antitrypsin glycogen storage
- Hemochromatosis in hereditary form
- Tyrosinemia with tardive porphyria cutanea
- Wilson's illness

How is liver cancer treated

For liver cancer, there are several therapy options. When proposing a course of therapy, your doctor will take into account many criteria. These consist of:

the quantity, size, and location of liver tumors, the health of your liver, the presence of cirrhosis, if cancer has migrated to other organs, and more. Among the liver cancer treatments are:

Partial Liver Removal

To remove a section of the liver, a partial hepatectomy is done. Only liver cancer in its early stages is routinely treated with this operation. The healthy tissue that is still there will eventually grow back and fill up the gap.

An Organ Transplant

During a liver transplant, the complete liver is swapped out with a healthy liver from a reliable donor. If the disease has not progressed to other organs, a transplant may be an option.

Following the transplant, you will be prescribed medicine to stop your body from rejecting the new liver.

Ablation

Ablation includes destroying the cancer cells using heat, cold, or ethanol injections. A local anesthetic is frequently used during the procedure. To keep you from experiencing pain, this numbs the region.

Ablation can help people who aren't candidates for surgery or a transplant.

Radiation therapy

Radiation therapy uses beams of high-energy radiation to kill cancer cells. It can be delivered by external beam radiation or by internal radiation.

In external beam radiation, the radiation is aimed at the parts of your body where cancer is located. Internal radiation involves the insertion of a small amount of radioactive material directly into or near cancer.

Targeted therapy

Targeted therapy uses medications designed to decrease tumor growth and blood supply. Compared to chemotherapy or radiation, these medications are fine-tuned to treat cancer cells only. This means that healthy cells can be spared from harm.

However, these medications can still cause serious side effects.

Targeted therapy can be helpful for people who aren't candidates for a hepatectomy or liver transplant. Medications of this type include tyrosine kinase inhibitors (TKIs), such as:
- cabozantinib (Cabometyx or Cometriq)
- lenvatinib (Lenvima)
- regorafenib (Stivarga)
- sorafenib (Nexavar)

Embolization, chemoembolization, and radioembolization.

Embolization procedures are used to reduce blood supply to liver tumors. Your doctor will insert small particles to create a partial blockage in the hepatic artery. This reduces the amount of blood flowing to the tumor. Another blood vessel known as the portal vein continues to nourish the healthy liver tissue.

In chemoembolization, your doctor injects chemotherapy drugs into the hepatic artery before injecting the blocking particles. This sends the chemotherapy drugs directly into the tumor. The blockage reduces blood flow to the tumor.

Radioembolization is a combination of radiation therapy and embolization. It involves injecting tiny radioactive beads into the hepatic artery. This decreases blood flow to the tumor and provides radiation therapy to the direct area of the tumor.

Chemotherapy

Chemotherapy is a powerful form of drug therapy that destroys cancer cells. The medications are typically injected intravenously or through a vein. In most cases, you can receive chemotherapy as an outpatient treatment.

Chemotherapy may be used for liver cancer when other therapies aren't appropriate or aren't working well. Because chemotherapy affects healthy cells in your body, not just the cancer cells, side effects are common.

Immunotherapy

Immunotherapy treats cancer using your body's immune system. Treatment with immunotherapy drugs can help your body recognize and destroy cancer cells. Like other cancer therapies, serious side effects are possible.

How can liver cancer be prevented?

You can't always prevent liver cancer. However, you can reduce your risk for liver cancer by taking steps to protect the health of your liver.

Get the hepatitis B vaccine

There's a vaccine for hepatitis B that is recommended for all eligible children. Adults who are at high risk for infection should also be vaccinated.

This includes people who use illegal drugs like heroin, crack cocaine, and crystal methamphetamine.

The vaccination is usually given in a series of three injections over 6 months.

Take measures to prevent hepatitis C

There's no vaccine for hepatitis C, but there are several ways to reduce the risk of getting the infection:

- Use condoms. You can reduce your risk of getting hepatitis by using a condom every time you have sex. If you and your partner are thinking about stopping condom use, it's important to talk with them first about getting tested for hepatitis and other sexually transmitted infections (STIs).

- Be aware of the hepatitis risk associated with illegal drug use. There's a high risk of hepatitis C infection among people who inject illegal drugs. To reduce hepatitis risk, those who use these drugs should use new, sterile equipment (like needles) every time. It's important not to share needles or other equipment with others. The best way to prevent hepatitis infection is to stop injecting.

- Be cautious about tattoos and piercings. Go to a trustworthy shop for a piercing or tattoo. Regulations on tattoo and piercing safety vary state by state, so check out the relevant laws and licensing in your area. Sterile and safe practices are very important, so it's best to make sure you're going to a shop that takes infection control seriously.

All types of hepatitis can be treated, and hepatitis C can sometimes be cured. If you test positive for hepatitis, it's important to talk with a doctor about treatment options.

Reduce your risk of cirrhosis

Changes you can make to lower your risk of cirrhosis include the following:

If you drink alcohol, drink in moderation.

Limiting the amount of alcohol you drink can help prevent liver damage. Because of the differences in how alcohol is processed in your body, moderate drinking guidelines differ by sex:

Female: up to one alcoholic drink per day
Male: up to two alcoholic drinks per day

Take steps to treat obesity
Obesity increases your risk of liver cancer. Obesity is associated with a higher risk of nonalcoholic fatty liver disease, which can lead to cirrhosis.
Talking with a doctor is a good way to determine lifestyle changes or other treatments for obesity.

Live a healthy lifestyle
Higher levels of physical activity may reduce your risk of liver cancer. Exercising regularly can improve your general health. It's also an important part of maintaining your weight within a healthier range.

Eating a balanced diet
Eating a balanced diet is important for cancer prevention. Make sure you incorporate lean protein, whole grains, and vegetables into your meals.

If being overweight or obese is a concern for you, talk with a doctor or dietician about creating a meal plan for healthy weight loss.

10. Kidney Cancer

The kidneys are two bean-shaped organs, each about the size of a fist. They're located in your abdomen on either side of your spine. The kidneys filter out waste from your blood and make urine. Different types of cancer can affect your kidneys.

The National Cancer Institute (NCI) estimates that there were more than 76,000 new cases of kidney cancer diagnosed in the United States in 2021, making up about 4 percent of all new cancers diagnosed for that year.

While the incidence of kidney cancer appears to be increasing, the NCI also notes a steadily decreasing death rate from this cancer. This may be possibly attributed to earlier detection, as well as new treatments.

Signs include:
- Blood in your urine
- Pain in one side of your lower back that isn't caused by an injury
- A lump on one side of your lower back
- Feeling tired all the time
- A low appetite
- Losing weight without trying
- A fever that doesn't go away
- Anemia (low red blood cell counts, which your doctor would determine with a blood test).

What are the types of kidney cancer?

Several types of cancer can affect the kidneys:

Renal cell carcinoma (RCC)

RCC is also known as renal cell adenocarcinoma. As many as 9 out of 10 kidney cancers are this type, making RCC the most common type of kidney cancer, according to the American Cancer Society (ACS). It starts in the part of the kidney that filters blood and usually involves a single tumor on one kidney.

It most commonly affects men ages 50 to 70.

Clear cell renal cell carcinoma

This RCC subtype makes up an estimated 7 out of 10 cases of RCC. It's called a "clear cell" due to the pale or clear appearance of the cells in a lab.

Non-clear cell renal cell carcinomas

This RCC subtype is rarer and doesn't appear clear under a microscope. Non-clear cell renal cell carcinomas include two types: papillary RCC and chromophobe RCC.

Renal pelvis carcinoma

Renal pelvis carcinoma starts in the part of the kidney where urine is collected.

Renal sarcoma

While not as common, renal sarcoma is a type of kidney cancer that starts in connective tissues or blood vessels.

Wilms' tumor

Wilms' tumor is considered a non-clear cell RCC. It is the most common type of kidney cancer in children under the age of 5 and may also occur in some adults.

Treatment options for kidney cancer

The treatment for kidney cancer focuses on removing the tumor from your body. This is usually done through surgery. Surgery can be radical or conservative.

However, metastatic kidney cancer — kidney cancer that has spread to other parts of the body — can't be treated with surgery alone. After as much tumor is removed as possible with surgery, other treatments may be necessary. These may include immunotherapy, targeted therapy, and radiation.

Radical nephrectomy

A radical nephrectomy is a surgical procedure that removes your kidney. The entire organ is removed, along with some surrounding tissue and lymph nodes. The adrenal gland may be removed as well. The surgery can be done through a large incision or with a laparoscope, which consists of a thin tube with a tiny camera at one end.

Conservative nephrectomy

Conservative nephrectomy removes only the tumor, lymph nodes, and some surrounding tissue. Part of the kidney is left behind. This is also known as a nephron-sparing nephrectomy. Tumor cells can also be destroyed by freezing, which is called cryosurgery, or radiofrequency ablation, which involves applying heat.

Radiation therapy

Radiation therapy may be used to damage or destroy cancer cells with high-energy waves. This may stop them from growing and spreading. Radiation is often performed to target cancer cells that may remain after surgery. It is considered a local treatment, which means it is often used for just a specific area of the body.

Chemotherapy

Chemotherapy is a chemical drug therapy used to treat cancer. It targets rapidly growing cancer cells and affects the whole body. It may be recommended by a doctor if cancer has spread, or metastasized, from the kidneys to other parts of the body.

Immunotherapy

Immunotherapy is a special treatment that helps your immune system recognize the cancer cells and fight cancer more effectively. Examples of immunotherapy used to treat kidney cancer include Pembrolizumab (Keytruda) and Nivolumab (Opdivo).

Targeted drugs

Targeted drugs are designed to block certain abnormal signals present in kidney cancer cells. They can help stop the formation of new blood vessels to supply nutrients to cancer cells.

Examples of targeted drugs include:

1. axitinib (Inlyta)
2. lenvatinib (Lenvima)

3. pazopanib (Votrient)
4. sorafenib (Nexavar)
5. sunitinib (Sutent)

Avoiding Kidney Cancer

The most effective strategy to lower your risk of kidney cancer is to lead a healthy lifestyle. You may take specific measures to lower your risk, such as:

- Not a smoker
- Maintaining a healthy diet
- Keeping at a healthy weight
- Defending oneself at work against toxic poisons
- Maintaining blood pressure management

11. Bone cancer

When a tumor, or abnormal mass of tissue, develops in a bone, bone cancer results. They are referred to as bone sarcomas.

A tumor may be malignant, meaning it is growing quickly and affecting other bodily components. It's common to describe a malignant tumor as cancerous.

Any bone in your body may develop into bone cancer, but it often does so in the pelvic bone or one of the long bones in your arms or legs, such as the shinbone, femur, or upper arm.

Bone cancer is a rare kind of cancer. It may, however, be aggressive, therefore early identification is crucial.

Bone cancer may also develop from cancer that started in another part of the body. Typically, cancer is called for the site where it first appears.

Types of Bone Cancers

The most dangerous types of bone cancer are primary ones. They develop immediately inside the bone or nearby tissue, like cartilage.

Additionally, cancer may metastasize, or spread, from another region of your body to your bones. This kind of bone cancer is called secondary bone cancer, and it is more prevalent than primary bone cancer.

Primary bone tumors of various forms include:

Osteosarcoma (osteogenic sarcoma)

Although it may affect adults, osteosarcoma, also known as osteogenic sarcoma, often affects children and adolescents. The points of long bones in the arms and legs are where it often begins to develop.

Besides the hips and shoulders, osteosarcoma may also develop in other places. It affects the bony tissue that makes up your bones' outer layer.

Two out of every three instances of primary bone cancer are osteosarcomas, which are the most prevalent kind.

Sarcoma of Ewing

The second most common primary bone cancer is Ewing's sarcoma. Children and young adults are often affected by this condition, which either starts in the soft tissues surrounding the bones or in the bones themselves.

The pelvic and long bones of your body, such as your arms and legs, are often impacted.

Chondrosarcoma

Older individuals' shoulders, thighs, and pelvis are where chondrosarcoma most often develops. The subchondral tissue, the strong connective tissue between your bones, is where it develops. These tumors often develop slowly. The least frequent primary cancer of the bones is this one.

Several myelomas

The most prevalent kind of cancer affecting the bones in multiple myeloma (MM).

However, since it starts in plasma cells, it is not regarded as primary bone cancer. Tumors develop in different bones as a result of the growth of cancerous cells in the bone marrow. MM often affects elderly people.

Staging And Diagnosis Of Bone Cancer

Primary bone cancer is staged by doctors. These many phases explain cancer's location, behavior, and extent of spread to other body parts:

1. The bone has not been invaded by stage 1 bone cancer.

2. Even though stage 2 bone cancer has not migrated to other tissues, it might become invasive.
3. Stage 3 bone cancer is invasive and has spread to one or more bone regions.
4. In stage 4 bone cancer, the disease has metastasized to nearby tissues and other organs including the lungs or brain.

The following techniques may be used by your doctor to ascertain the stage of bone cancer:

Biopsy

A biopsy determines if cancer is present by examining a tiny sample of tissue.

a bone scan that examines the health of the bones

a blood test to provide a baseline for use in the course of therapy imaging tests such as X-rays, PET, MRI, and CT scans to gain detailed pictures of the bone structure

Grading

Following a biopsy, doctors may grade tumors according to how they appear under a microscope. Based on how much they resemble regular cells, the grade serves as a gauge of how likely it is that they will develop and spread.

Typically, the more abnormal they seem, the quicker they could spread and expand. There are two grades of bone cancer: low grade and high grade.

A higher grade may indicate that the cells are more atypical and are likely to spread more quickly, while a lower grade may indicate that the cells are more normal and are likely to spread more slowly.

Doctors may choose the best course of therapy with the aid of the grade.

Bone Cancer Treatment

Treatment is based on:

- Cancer's grade and stage.
- Your age and general well-being.
- The tumor's dimensions and location.

Medications

The following drugs are used to treat bone cancer:

- Chemotherapeutic medicines for MM.
- Analgesics to reduce pain and inflammation.
- Bisphosphonates to maintain bone structure and stop bone loss.
- To prevent or halt the development of malignant cells, use cytotoxic medicines.
- medicines used in immunotherapy to boost the body's defenses against cancer cells.

Surgery

Tumors or damaged tissue may be surgically removed by a doctor. One way to avoid cancer from spreading fast is via surgery to remove damaged bone and replace it.

Amputation may be required if the arms or legs have a severe bone injury.

Radiation Treatment

Radiation treatment may be suggested by a doctor to eradicate cancer cells. To limit the proliferation of cancer cells, this therapy may be used in combination with another kind of treatment.

If surgery is unable to remove enough of the tumor, radiation therapy may also be utilized.

Complementary Medicine

Your care plan could also involve other therapies that include herbal remedies, according to the doctor. This must be done carefully, however, since certain complementary therapies could conflict with chemotherapy and radiation therapy.

The use of complementary treatments may help you feel better overall and experience symptom alleviation. Other alternatives include:
meditation, yoga and aromatherapy.

12. Myeloma Cancer

Multiple myeloma is a kind of cancer that arises when an abnormal plasma cell grows and multiplies rapidly in the bone marrow. Eventually, the creation of healthy cells in the bone marrow is surpassed by the myeloma cancer cells' fast cell division.

Monoclonal (M) proteins are abnormal antibodies produced by malignant myeloma cells that have the potential to harm the kidneys and other vital organs.

It's uncommon to have multiple myeloma. The National Cancer Institute predicts that there will be 34,920 new cases of multiple myeloma in the United States in 2021. That represents around 1.8% of all new cancer cases.

Multiple Myeloma Types

Multiple myeloma may be of two basic types:

Idiopathic Myeloma. This kind often takes a long time to manifest any symptoms. Only little increases in M protein and M plasma cells occur, not bone cancers.

Individual Plasmacytoma. This kind often causes a tumor to develop in the bone. Although it normally responds favorably to therapy, it requires watchful observation.

How is multiple myeloma handled medically?

No treatment exists for multiple myeloma. There are, however, medical procedures that may lessen discomfort, lessen problems, and halt the spread of the illness. Only when the condition is growing worse are treatments administered.

If you don't have any symptoms, your doctor is not likely to recommend therapy. Instead, your medical professional will carefully watch for symptoms of a developing illness. Frequently, this entails routine urine and blood tests.
If you want medical attention, the following are typical options:

Targeted treatment
Targeted treatment drugs prevent a chemical from destroying proteins in myeloma cells and killing the cancer cells.
During targeted treatment, medications such as bortezomib (Velcade) and carfilzomib may be used (Kyprolis). Both medicines are injected directly into a vein in your arm.

Medical treatment
Drugs used in biological treatment target myeloma cells with the immune system of your

body. Immune system boosters like thalidomide (Thalomid), lenalidomide (Revlimid), and pomalidomide (Pomalyst) are often taken as pills.

Though lenalidomide has fewer negative effects than thalidomide, they are comparable. It also seems to be stronger.

Chemotherapy

Chemotherapy is an intensive pharmacological treatment that aids in the destruction of rapidly proliferating cells, such as myeloma cells. High dosages of chemotherapy medications are often used, particularly before a stem cell transplant. The drugs may be administered intravenously or ingested as pills.

Corticosteroids

Prednisone and dexamethasone are two corticosteroids that are often used to treat myeloma. They often work well in eliminating myeloma cells because they may regulate the immune system by lowering inflammatory levels in the body. They may be administered intravenously or as pills.

Radiation Treatment

Strong energy beams are used in radiation treatment to harm myeloma cells and halt their proliferation. This kind of therapy is sometimes used to swiftly eliminate myeloma cells in a specific location of the body.

For instance, it could be carried out when a plasmacytoma, a painful tumor made up of abnormal plasma cells, breaks down bone.

Transplantation of stem cells

In stem cell transplants, healthy bone marrow is used to replace damaged bone marrow. Allogenic stem cells from a donor or your stem cells are what create healthy bone marrow (autologous).

Blood-forming stem cells are taken from the patient's blood before the surgery. After that, high-dose chemotherapy or radiation treatment is used to treat multiple myeloma.

The stem cells may be injected into your body after the damaged tissue has been removed, at which point they travel into the bones and begin to regenerate bone marrow.

Complementary medicine

The use of complementary medicine, also known as integrative medicine, has grown in popularity as a means of easing multiple myeloma symptoms and treatment side effects.

Although these treatments cannot treat or cure multiple myeloma, they could help you feel better.

Before implementing any of these treatments, discuss them with your doctor. Make sure they are appropriate for you and your current health situation. Acupuncture, aromatherapy, massage, meditation, and relaxation techniques are possible forms of treatment.

13. Cervical Cancer

One kind of cancer that begins in the cervix is cervical cancer. The bottom portion of a woman's uterus is connected to her vagina through a hollow tube called the cervix. Cells on the cervix's surface are where the majority of cervical cancers start.

In the past, American women's deaths from cervical cancer were among the most common. However, since screening tests became readily accessible, things have altered.

Cervical Cancer Signs And Symptoms

Because cervical cancer often doesn't present symptoms until later stages, many women with the illness are unaware of their condition when it first arises. When symptoms do emerge, they might easily be confused with common diseases like menstruation and urinary tract infections (UTIs).

- Unusual bleeding, such as between periods, after sex, or after menopause.
- Vaginal discharge that looks or smells different from normal.
- Discomfort in the pelvis.
- Having to pee more often.

- Pain while urinating is typical of cervical cancer symptoms.

Visit your doctor for a checkup if you experience any of these symptoms.

Causes Of Cervical Cancer

The sexually transmitted **Human Papillomavirus** is the primary factor in most occurrences of cervical cancer (HPV). Genital warts are brought on by the same virus.

There are over 100 distinct HPV strains. *Cervical cancer is only caused by certain kinds. HPV-16 and HPV-18 are the two strains that cause cancer the most often.*

Cervical cancer is not a guarantee even if you have an HPV cancer-causing strain. Most HPV infections are cleared up by your immune system, often within two years.

1. In both men and women, HPV may lead to other malignancies. Among them is vulvar cancer.
2. uterine cancer
3. prostate cancer
4. throat cancer
5. throat cancer, rectal cancer

Carcinoma Of The Cervix Therapy

If detected early, cervical cancer is highly curable. The four primary therapies are as follows:

- Surgery
- Radiation treatment
- Chemotherapy
- Targeted treatment

These therapies are sometimes combined to increase their potency.

Surgery

The goal of surgery is to eradicate as much cancer as is humanly feasible. The doctor may sometimes be able to remove just the portion of the cervix that has cancerous cells. The cervix and other pelvic organs may need to be removed during surgery for more advanced malignancy.

Radiation Treatment

X-ray beams with high energy are used in radiation to destroy cancer cells. It may be given by a device outside the body. A metal tube inserted into the uterus or vagina may also be used to deliver it from inside the body.

Chemotherapy

Drugs are used in chemotherapy to eradicate cancer cells throughout the body. This therapy is cycled via doctors. You'll undergo chemotherapy for a while. After then, the therapy will end so that your body has time to heal.

Targeted treatment

A more recent medication called bevacizumab (Avastin) functions differently from chemotherapy and radiation. Inhibiting the development of new blood vessels prevents the tumor from spreading and surviving. Often, this medication is used together with chemotherapy.

Stages Of Cervical Cancer

Your doctor will determine the stage of your cancer when a diagnosis has been made. The stage reveals if and how far cancer has spread if it has. Your doctor can identify the best course of therapy for you by staging your cancer.

Four phases of cervical cancer exist:

Stage 1: Little cancer. There's a chance the lymph nodes were affected. It hasn't spread to other bodily areas.

Stage 2: The tumor has grown. It can have reached the lymph nodes or spread beyond the uterus and cervix. It hasn't yet spread to other areas of your body.

Stage 3: The malignancy has gone to the pelvic or the lower vagina. The ureters, which are tubes that transfer urine from the kidneys to the bladder, may be blocked as a result. It hasn't spread to other bodily areas.

Stage 4: The disease may have gone to your lungs, bones, or liver in addition to your pelvis.

Prevention Of Cervical Cancer.

Regular Pap smear or hrHPV testing is one of the simplest methods to screen for cervical cancer. Precancerous cells are detected during screening so they may be treated before they progress to malignancy.

Most occurrences of cervical cancer are caused by HPV infection. With the help of the vaccinations Gardasil and Cervarix, the illness may be avoided. The best time for vaccination is before a person starts acting sexually. Boys and girls may both get the HPV vaccine.

You may lessen your risk of HPV and cervical cancer by doing the following additional things:
Reduce the number of people you have sex with, and if you have vaginal, oral, or anal intercourse, always use a condom or other barrier device.

14. Duodenal cancer

The first and tiniest section of the small intestine is called the duodenum. It is situated halfway through your small intestine, between your stomach and the jejunum. The horseshoe-shaped duodenum takes food from the stomach that hasn't been fully digested.

In the digestive process, this organ is crucial. To aid in breaking down food that has been passed from the stomach, bile and chemical secretions are discharged into the duodenum. Before the meal is transported to the jejunum, vitamins and other nutrients start to be absorbed into the body here.

Even though it is uncommon, duodenal cancer may interfere with this digestive process and stop your body from receiving vital minerals.

Signs Of Duodenal Cancer

An uncommon kind of cancer of the digestive system is duodenal cancer. Tumors may prevent food from entering the digestive system when cancer cells start to grow in the duodenum.

You may suffer a multitude of symptoms when food cannot pass through the small intestine or when the body cannot absorb vital vitamins:

1. cramps in the stomach

2. nausea
3. constipation
4. vomiting
5. acid retching
6. slim down
7. soiled stools

The majority of the time, duodenal cancer symptoms don't show up until the illness has progressed to the point where the tumor is big enough to restrict the passage of food. You could then detect an abdominal lump.

Duodenal Cancer Types
Adenocarcinoma

The glandular cells that produce mucus, digestive enzymes and other body fluids from internal organs are impacted by this kind of cancer.

Sarcoma

A sarcoma is a particular kind of malignant tumor that develops in the body's fat, blood vessels, muscle, or soft tissues like bone.

Lymphoma
This form of cancer affects the immune system.

Stromal tumor of the digestive system
The walls of the gastrointestinal (GI) tract develop tumors from this malignancy.

Carcinoid growths
This kind of cancer's tumors often develop in the gastrointestinal tract and may result in carcinoid syndrome. They may also spread to other body parts and organs.

Therapy For Duodenal Cancer
Depending on the stage at which it was discovered, this uncommon cancer is treated differently. However, surgery alone or in combination with chemotherapy, radiation, or both is the most popular and efficient form of treatment.

To enable food to flow from the stomach, doctors will attempt to remove tumors from the duodenum. The Whipple technique, which also involves surgery, removes the duodenum, gallbladder, and a part of the pancreas.

Chemotherapy may be used as a substitute for surgery to eradicate dangerous cancer cells. However, this therapy has a variety of potential negative effects, such as: hair loss, nausea, and tiredness, as well as weight loss

Some individuals choose to get more holistic medical care, often including herbs and home medicines in their daily regimen. Some herbal treatments may lessen malignant tumors and alleviate painful symptoms. If you do wish to attempt utilizing such therapies, speak with your doctor first. They could have recommendations for things to try or worry about any drug interactions you might have.

CHAPTER THREE

15. Cancer Of The Ear

Both the internal and external components of the ear may be affected by ear cancer. It often begins as an ear skin carcinoma on the outer lobe and subsequently spreads to the eardrum, ear canal, and other ear structures.

Additionally, ear cancer may develop within the ear. The temporal bone, which is located within the ear, may be impacted. The mastoid bone is a part of the temporal bone. This is the bony bump behind your ear that you feel.

It is quite uncommon to have ear cancer. Only approximately 300 Americans get a diagnosis for it each year. On the other hand, the National Cancer Institute predicts that in 2018, there will be more than 250,000 new instances of breast cancer.

Various Ear Cancers.

The ear may be impacted by several cancer kinds. They consist of the following:

Skin Tumors

- The basal layer cells of the epidermis, or top layer of skin, are impacted by basal cell carcinoma.
- The squamous cells of the epidermis are impacted by squamous cell cancer. The most common kind of ear cancer is this one. It penetrates the body's cells more deeply and has a higher propensity than basal cell carcinoma to spread to other tissues. According to a 2016 case study, squamous cell carcinomas that damage the outer cartilage of the ear have a 15% probability of disseminating.
- Melanoma affects the melanocyte cells of the skin. When exposed to the sun, these cells turn the skin brown. Melanoma is a more dangerous kind of skin cancer than basal or squamous cell carcinoma, although being less prevalent. It is

regarded as the most dangerous kind of skin cancer. According to a 2006 analysis, 1% of occurrences of melanoma are ear-related.

Cystic Adenoid Carcinoma

Although it primarily affects the salivary glands, this very uncommon kind of cancer may also develop in the ear. According to a 2013 case study, these tumors make up just 5% of malignancies of the external auditory canal (the passageway from the outside of the head to the eardrum).

Parotid Tumors

The ear canal may get infected by parotid gland cancerous growths. The biggest salivary gland in the body is this one.

Symptoms Of Ear Cancer

Depending on which portion of your ear is damaged, different ear cancer symptoms may be present.

Outside Ear

The earlobe, ear rim (sometimes known as the pinna), and outer ear canal entrance are all parts of the outer ear.

Outer ear skin cancer warning signs include:

After moisturizing pearly white lumps beneath the skin, scaly areas of the skin persist, bleeding skin ulcers

Ear Canal

Hearing loss, a mass at or near the ear canal's entrance, and an ear discharge are all indications of skin cancer in the ear canal.

Center Ear

Middle ear skin cancer warning signs include:

- An ear discharge that may be bloody (most common symptom)
- loss of hearing
- numbness on the afflicted side of the head and discomfort in the ears

Inside ear

- Inner ear skin cancer symptoms include:
- Ears hurt
- Dizziness
- Headache ringing in the ears.
- Hearing loss

Ear Cancer Causes

What specifically causes ear cancer is unknown. Because there are so few occurrences, it's difficult to guess where it could have come from. However, scientists are aware that a few factors may make you more likely to get ear cancer. These consist of:

1. Having fair skin. This raises your overall chance of developing skin cancer.
2. Being exposed to the sun without using enough (or any) sunscreen. You are more likely to get skin cancer as a result, which may cause ear cancer.
3. Having ear infections often. Ear infections' inflammatory reactions may potentially affect the cellular alterations that lead to cancer.

4. Growing older. Age is a factor in the prevalence of several ear cancer forms. According to data from one research, the seventh decade of life is when squamous cell carcinoma of the temporal bone is most frequent.

Therapy For Ear Cancer

The size and location of the malignant tumor are the main determinants of treatment.

On the exterior of the ear, skin malignancies are often removed. You could need reconstructive surgery if substantial sections are removed.

Cancers of the temporal bone or ear canal need radiation treatment after surgery. The size of the tumor determines how much of the ear must be removed.

Sometimes it's necessary to remove the eardrum, bone, and canal. Your doctor may be able to repair your ear depending on how much is removed.

Hearing isn't always greatly impacted. You may need to wear a hearing aid in other situations.

16. Endometrial Cancer

Uterine cancer that begins in the uterus's inner lining is known as endometrial cancer. The endometrium is the term for this lining.

The National Cancer Institute (NCI) estimates that 3 out of 100 women may get a uterine cancer diagnosis at some time in their life. After being diagnosed with uterine cancer, more than 80% of patients live for five years or longer.

Your chances of going into remission if you have endometrial cancer are increased by early detection and treatment.

What Signs Indicate Endometrial Cancer?

Abnormal vaginal bleeding is one of endometrial cancer's most prevalent symptoms. This may consist of:

- alterations in the duration or intensity of menstrual cycles
- spotting or bleeding in the cervix between menstrual cycles
- bleeding in the vagina after menopause

The following are other signs of endometrial cancer:

- Discomfort in the lower abdomen or pelvis during intercourse
- Watery or bloody vaginal discharge
- Unexpected weight loss

Make an appointment with your doctor if you notice any of these signs. Even while these symptoms do not always indicate a significant problem, it's still vital to get them examined.

Menopause or other noncancerous diseases may result in abnormal vaginal bleeding. But sometimes, it's a symptom of gynecological cancer, such as endometrial cancer.

If necessary, your doctor can suggest the best course of action and assist you in determining the origin of your problems.

What kinds of endometrial cancer are there?

According to the ACS, adenocarcinomas, which are cancers that arise from glandular tissue, account for the majority of occurrences of endometrial cancer.

Endometrial cancer may take on less typical forms, such as:

- Carcinosarcoma of the womb (CS)
- carcinoma of the squamous cell
- crossover carcinoma
- Serous cancer

There are two basic categories into which endometrial carcinoma may be divided:

- Type 1 usually develops slowly and doesn't immediately spread to other tissues.
- Type 2 is more likely to expand beyond the uterus and tends to be more aggressive.

Compared to type 2, type 1 endometrial cancers are more prevalent. Also, they are simpler to heal.

What therapies are available to treat endometrial cancer?

There are several endometrial cancer treatments available. The course of therapy that your doctor advises will depend on the subtype and stage of your cancer, as well as your general health and preferences.

Each treatment option has potential advantages and disadvantages.

Surgery

Hysterectomy surgery is often used to treat endometrial cancer.

A hysterectomy involves the removal of the uterus by a surgeon. They may also perform a technique called a bilateral salpingo-oophorectomy in which the ovaries and fallopian tubes are removed (BSO). BSO and hysterectomy are often carried out together.

The surgeon will also take out any adjacent lymph nodes to determine whether cancer has spread. This is referred to as lymphadenectomy or lymph node dissection.

Radiation Treatment

High-energy beams are used in radiation treatment to eliminate cancer cells.

To treat endometrial cancer, radiation treatment is primarily divided into two categories:

Radiation treatment using an external beam: Radiation beams are focused on the uterus by a piece of equipment outside of your body.

Treatment with internal radiation: The vagina or uterus is given radioactive elements to put within the body. This also goes by the name of brachytherapy.

After surgery, your doctor can suggest either one or both forms of radiation treatment. This may aid in the elimination of any cancer cells that could survive the surgery.

In exceptional circumstances, they could advise radiation treatment before surgery. Tumors may get smaller, as a result, making removal simpler.

Your doctor could suggest radiation therapy as your primary treatment if you are unable to have surgery owing to other medical issues or poor general health.

Chemotherapy

Chemotherapy uses medication to eradicate cancer cells. A single medicine may be used in certain chemotherapy treatments, whereas many drugs may be used in others. The medications may be either orally or intravenously, depending on the kind of chemotherapy you get.

If your endometrial cancer has spread to other body sites or has come back after previous treatment, your doctor may advise chemotherapy.

Immunotherapy and targeted treatment

The use of medications designed to target specific alterations in the cancer cells is a relatively recent method of treating endometrial cancer. Since many of these targeted treatment medications are still being tested in clinical studies, only a small number of them are now on the market.

Another more customized method is immunotherapy, which is administering medicines to help your immune system identify and eliminate cancer cells.

There are times when chemotherapy and immunotherapy are combined, as well as targeted medicines.

hormone treatment

Hormone treatment modifies the body's hormone levels by using hormones or hormone-blocking medications. Endometrial cancer cells may develop more slowly as a result.

Hormone treatment may be suggested by your doctor if you have stage III or stage IV endometrial cancer. Additionally, if endometrial cancer has returned after therapy, they could advise it.

Chemotherapy is often paired with hormone treatment.

Emotional Assistance

Inform your doctor if you're experiencing emotional difficulties dealing with your cancer diagnosis or treatment. People often struggle to control the emotional and mental repercussions of having cancer.

Your doctor may suggest that you join a local or online cancer support group. Connecting with others who are experiencing similar things as you could be reassuring.

Your physician could suggest that you seek therapy from a mental health professional. You may be able to handle the psychological and social repercussions of having cancer with the support of one-on-one or group therapy.

Esophagus or Throat Cancer

The esophagus, a muscular hollow tube, transports food from the neck to the stomach. A malignant growth may develop in the lining of the esophagus, which can lead to esophageal cancer.

The muscle and deep tissues of the esophagus may be affected when the tumor spreads. Anywhere along the length of the esophagus, including the junction with the stomach, might develop a tumor.

What are the types of esophageal cancer?

Esophageal cancer often comes in two different forms:

- When cancer begins in the flat, flimsy cells that make up the lining of the esophagus, squamous cell carcinoma develops. This type may develop anywhere in the esophagus, however, it often develops at the top or center.

- When cancer begins in the esophageal glandular cells that produce mucus and other fluids, such as adenocarcinoma develops. The lower part of the esophagus is where adenocarcinomas are most often seen.

What Signs Indicate Esophageal Cancer?
You most likely won't have any symptoms in the early stages of esophageal cancer. You can encounter the following when your cancer worsens:
1. Indigestion.
2. Unintended weight loss.
3. Chest discomfort.
4. Weariness.
5. A persistent cough.
6. Hiccups, heartburn, pain or trouble swallowing.
7. Often choking while eating.

8. Vomiting.

9. Food coming back up the esophagus.

Esophageal Cancer Treatment

Depending on whether cancer has spread to other areas of your body, your doctor may advise surgery.

As an alternative, your doctor could advise chemotherapy or radiation treatment as the best course of action. To make esophageal tumor removal during surgery easier, these therapies are sometimes used to reduce the size of the tumors.

Surgery

Your doctor may remove the tumor with a minimally invasive procedure if the cancer is small and hasn't spread using an endoscope and a few tiny incisions.

The surgeon uses the conventional technique to remove a section of the esophagus and sometimes the lymph nodes around it via a bigger incision. With tissue from the stomach or large intestine, the tube is rebuilt.

In extreme circumstances, the top of the stomach could also need to be removed in part.

The potential side effects of surgery may include discomfort, bleeding, infection, lung difficulties, trouble swallowing, nausea, and heartburn. They can also include leakage where the reconstructed esophagus connects to the stomach.

Chemotherapy

Drugs are used in chemotherapy to target cancer cells. Surgery may be performed either before or after chemotherapy. It sometimes happens when radiation treatment is used.

There are several potential negative effects of chemotherapy. Most occur as a result of chemotherapy medicines that also destroy healthy cells. The medications your doctor employs will have an impact on your side effects. These negative impacts may consist of: hair loss, indigestion, lethargy, discomfort, and neuropathy

Radiation Treatment

To eliminate cancer cells, radiation treatment employs radiation beams. Radiation may be delivered either inside or externally (via a machine) (with a device placed near the tumor, which is called brachytherapy).

Chemotherapy and radiation are often combined, and the adverse effects are typically more severe. Radiation side effects might include:

- skin that seems sunburned
- esophageal lining ulcers that are unpleasant and cause difficulties swallowing

Long after the end of the therapy, certain adverse effects may still be felt. These include esophageal stricture, in which the tissue loses flexibility and may restrict the esophagus, causing discomfort or making swallowing difficult.

Targeted Treatment.

Specific proteins on cancer cells may be targeted by targeted medicines to treat the disease.

Trastuzumab may be used to treat a small percentage of esophageal malignancies. It targets the HER2 protein on the cancer cell's surface, where the protein has been promoting the growth of the cancer cells.

Cancers may also develop new blood vessels to grow and spread. Ramucirumab, a kind of "monoclonal antibody" targeted treatment, binds to the VEGF protein, which promotes the growth of new blood vessels.

Esophageal Cancer Prevention
Esophageal cancer cannot be completely avoided, however, there are certain things you can do to reduce your risk:
1. The secret is avoiding chewing tobacco and cigarettes.
2. It is also believed that limiting your alcohol intake would reduce your risk.
3. Esophageal cancer may also be prevented by eating a diet high in fruits and vegetables and keeping a healthy weight.

17. Cancer of the heart

The heart may develop abnormal growths called primary cardiac tumors. They are unusual. Less than 1 in 2000 autopsies, according to the European Society of Cardiology (ESC), include them.

Primary cardiac tumors may be cancerous or noncancerous (benign) (malignant). While benign tumors don't metastasize, malignant tumors do develop into adjacent tissues or spread to other areas of the body. Primary cardiac tumors are mostly benign. Only 25%, according to the ESC, are malignant.

Secondary heart cancer is cancer that has metastasized or spread from other organs to the heart. The ESC states that while it is currently very rare, it may happen up to 40 times more often than primary cardiac malignancies.

The most common cancers that metastasize or spread to the heart are:
- lung disease
- melanoma (skin cancer)

- mammary cancer
- renal cancer

lymphoma and leukemia (this is different than primary cardiac lymphoma in that it starts in the lymph nodes, spleen, or bone marrow instead of the heart)

Cancer Of The Heart Signs

Primary heart cancer symptoms may be divided into five groups.

1. An restriction on blood flow.

Blood flow through the heart may be obstructed when a tumor extends into one of the heart chambers or through a heart valve. Depending on where the tumor is, the symptoms might change

Atrium: A tumor in an upper heart chamber might resemble tricuspid or mitral valve stenosis by obstructing blood flow into the lower chambers (ventricles). You could experience this, particularly while exerting yourself, and feel out of breath and exhausted.

Ventricle: A tumor in a ventricle may imitate aortic or pulmonary valve stenosis by obstructing blood flow out of the heart. Chest discomfort, lightheadedness, weariness, and shortness of breath may all result from this.

2. Heart muscle impairment

Heart tumors may resemble cardiomyopathy or heart failure by growing into the heart's muscular walls, making them rigid and unable to pump blood efficiently. Some signs might be:

- breathing difficulty
- enlarged legs
- chest pain weakened exhaustion

3. Conducting issues

The rate and regularity of the heartbeat may be affected, resembling arrhythmias, by tumors that develop within the heart muscle near the conduction system. The natural conduction route between the atria and ventricles is often blocked by them. We refer to this as heart block. It indicates that rather than cooperating, the atria and ventricles independently establish their rhythm.

Depending on how severe it is, you could not even detect it or have a sluggish or skipped heartbeat. You can pass out or get exhausted if it moves too slowly. Ventricular fibrillation and abrupt cardiac arrest may result if the ventricles begin to beat quickly on their own.

4. Embolus

A blood clot or a small tumor fragment that breaks off and travels from the heart to another region of the body may lodge in a tiny artery. Depending on where the embolus lodges, different symptoms may appear:

Lung: Breathing difficulties, severe chest discomfort, and an erratic heartbeat may all be signs of a pulmonary embolism.

Brain: An embolic stroke often results in disorientation, difficulty speaking or understanding spoken or written words, weakness or paralysis on one side of the body, and a one-sided face droop.

Leg or arm: A limb affected by an artery embolism may become numb, uncomfortable, and chilly.

5. Generalized symptoms

Some primary cardiac tumors might present with vague symptoms that resemble infections. These signs might consist of:

- chills and a fever
- drowsiness night sweats
- loss of weight joint discomfort

The lining around the exterior of the heart is often invaded by the metastatic lesions of secondary heart cancer (pericardium). As a result, a malignant pericardial effusion—an accumulation of fluid surrounding the heart—is often caused.

The heart is pushed upon as the fluid level rises, which lowers the quantity of blood it can pump. Shortness of breath and sharp chest discomfort as you breathe in are symptoms, particularly when you're lying down.

When the heart is under extreme strain, little or no blood is pumped. The name of this potentially fatal disorder is cardiac tamponade. Arrhythmias, shock, and cardiac arrest may result from it.

Heart Cancer Causes

Why some individuals get heart cancer and others do not is a mystery to doctors. Few variables are known to increase the likelihood of developing certain kinds of cardiac tumors:

- Age: Some tumors are more common in adults, whereas others are more common in infants and young children.
- Heredity: Some of them may run in families.
- cancer syndromes caused by genes. Most kids with rhabdomyomas have tubular sclerosis, a disease brought on by a DNA mutation.
- immune system damage The majority of cases of primary cardiac lymphoma are

seen in patients with compromised immune systems.

- Contrary to pleural mesothelioma, which develops in the lining (mesothelium) of the lung, there is no known link between pericardial mesothelioma and asbestos exposure.

Choices For Heart Cancer Treatment

For all primary cardiac tumors, surgical removal is the preferred course of action.

Benign Tumors

If the tumor can be entirely removed, the majority of patients can be treated.

Removing a portion of a tumor that isn't within the heart walls may alleviate or improve symptoms in cases when there are many tumors or a huge tumor.

If they aren't producing symptoms, several kinds may be monitored with annual echocardiograms rather than surgery.

Malignant Tumors

They may be very challenging to treat since they spread quickly and infiltrate critical cardiac tissues.

Unfortunately, most don't get discovered until it's too late for surgical removal.

Palliative care practices include the use of chemotherapy and radiation therapy, however, these treatments are generally unsuccessful in treating primary heart cancer.

Secondary Heart Cancer

The disease has often progressed to other organs by the time cardiac metastases are discovered and is generally incurable.

The heart's metastatic illness cannot be surgically removed.

Often, the only choice is palliative care with chemotherapy and radiation treatment.

It is possible to drain a pericardial effusion if it forms by inserting a needle or tiny drain into the fluid accumulation (pericardiocentesis).

18. Gallbladder Cancer.

Under your liver, there is a little sac-like organ called the gallbladder that is roughly 3 inches long and 1 inch broad. Its function is to store bile, a fluid produced by your liver. Bile is discharged into your small intestine to aid in food digestion after being stored in your gallbladder.

Gallbladder cancer is uncommon. The American Cancer Society (ACS) reports:
In the United States, little over 12,000 persons will be diagnosed in 2019.

Adenocarcinoma, a kind of cancer that develops in glandular cells in the lining of your organs, is virtually invariably the cause.

Gallbladder Cancer Symptoms And Signs
Gallbladder cancer often doesn't show any signs until it's well advanced. Because of this, when it is discovered, it has often already migrated to neighboring lymph nodes and organs or other regions of your body.

When they do, here are some possible indications and symptoms:

- Pain in your belly, commonly in the upper right corner.
- When your bile ducts are blocked, you get jaundice, which is characterized by a yellowing of the skin and the whites of your eyes.
- Lumpy abdomen, which develops in the upper right abdomen when cancer progresses to the liver or your gallbladder enlarges as a result of clogged bile ducts.
- vomiting and nauseous.
- Loss of weight.
- Fever.
- stomach bloating
- tarry urine

Cancer Of The Gallbladder Treatment

Gallbladder cancer may be treated surgically, but only if all of the malignancy is removed. Only when the cancer is discovered early, before it has spread to surrounding organs and other areas of the body, is this a viable alternative.

Only approximately 1 in 5 persons, according to ACS data, get a diagnosis before the disease has progressed.

After surgery, chemotherapy and radiation are often used to ensure that all cancer has been removed. Additionally, it is used in the treatment of incurable gallbladder cancer. Cancer cannot be cured, but it may be managed and its symptoms treated.

Even with advanced gallbladder cancer, surgery is still an option for symptom relief. Palliative care is what this entails. Other forms of palliative care can consist of:

- Putting a tube, or stent, in the bile duct to keep it open so that it can drain
- pain medicine
- nausea medication
- oxygen

Palliative care is also used when a patient is too ill to undergo surgery.

Preventing Cancer Of The Gallbladder

Gallbladder cancer cannot be avoided since the majority of risk factors, such as age and ethnicity, cannot be altered. A healthy lifestyle, nevertheless, may help you reduce your risk. Here are some pointers for leading a healthy lifestyle:

- The maintenance of a healthy weight. This is a significant component of living a healthy lifestyle and one of the key strategies for reducing your chance of developing many cancers, including gallbladder cancer.

- Consuming a balanced diet. Consuming fruits and vegetables help strengthen your immune system and keep you healthy. You may maintain your health by eating whole grains rather than refined grains and avoiding processed meals.

- Exercising. Reaching and maintaining a healthy weight and bolstering your immune system are two advantages of moderate exercise.

19. Kidney Cancer

Two bean-shaped organs, the kidneys are each roughly the size of a hand. On each side of your spine, they are in your abdomen. Your kidneys produce urine and filter waste from your blood. Your kidneys may be impacted by a variety of cancers.

According to predictions from the National Cancer Institute (NCI), more than 76,000 new cases of kidney cancer were identified in the country in 2021, accounting for nearly 4% of all new cancer cases.

The NCI reports that the mortality rate from kidney cancer is consistently decreasing even though the incidence of the disease seems to be rising. This could be related to novel therapies as well as early diagnosis.

Kidney Cancer Symptoms And Signs

Early kidney cancer, when the tumor is tiny, often exhibits no symptoms. The signs and symptoms of cancer might include:

1. A backache that doesn't go away, particularly behind the ribs
2. pee with blood
3. a low back ache
4. weariness or a bump in your lower back or side
5. persistent fevers
6. reduced appetite
7. Anemia and unexplained weight loss

Why Does Kidney Cancer Develop?

There are various risk factors for kidney cancer, however, no recognized causes are specific.

What is known about how kidney cancer develops is that it follows a similar pattern to how other cancers develop, starting with aberrant cells in the body that proliferate and form tumors.

The location where cancers initially appear is also the source of their names. As a result, kidney cancer begins in the kidneys before spreading to other parts of the body.

What Forms Of Kidney Cancer Are There?

The kidneys may be impacted by many different cancers:

Cancer Of The Renal Cells (RCC)

Renal cell adenocarcinoma is an additional name for RCC. According to the American Cancer Society, RCC is the most prevalent kind of kidney cancer, accounting for up to 9 out of 10 cases (ACS). It often includes a single tumor on one kidney and begins in the portion of the kidney responsible for filtering blood.

Men from 50 to 70 years old are most often affected.

Renal cell carcinoma with clear cells

According to estimates, 7 out of 10 RCC instances belong to this subtype. Due to the cells' pale or transparent appearance in a lab, it is also known as "clear cell."

Renal Cell Carcinomas Without clear cells

Under a microscope, this RCC subtype is less common and doesn't seem clear. Papillary RCC and chromophobe RCC are two forms of non-clear cell renal cell carcinomas.

Kidney Pelvis Cancer

The area of the kidney where urine is stored is where renal pelvis cancer first appears.

Kidney Sarcoma

Renal sarcoma is a kind of kidney cancer that begins in connective tissues or blood vessels, although being less prevalent.

Cancer Of Wilms

Wilms' tumor is categorized as an RCC with non-clear cells. It may also happen to certain people. It is the most common kind of kidney cancer among kids under the age of five.

There are many unusual forms of kidney cancer, including:
- Multilocular RCC
- Collecting duct cystic RCC
- Medullary cancer linked with neuroblastoma

- Spindle cell
- Mucinous tubular carcinoma

Choices For Renal Cancer Treatment

The goal of kidney cancer therapy is to get the tumor out of your body. Surgery is often used to do this. Radical or conservative surgery is also possible.

However, surgery alone cannot cure kidney cancer that has metastasized or spread to other regions of the body. Other therapies can be required after the operation to eliminate the tumor as much as feasible. Radiation-targeted treatment and immunotherapy are a few examples.

Radical Kidney Removal

Your kidney is surgically removed during radical nephrectomy. Along with part of the surrounding tissue and lymph nodes, the whole organ is taken out. Additionally, the adrenal gland could be taken out. A major incision may be made during the procedure or a laparoscope, a slender tube with a microscopic camera at one end, can be used.

A Minimally Invasive Nephrectomy

Only the tumor, lymph nodes, and part of the surrounding tissue are removed with a conservative nephrectomy. The kidney is just partially removed. Nephron-sparing nephrectomy is another name for this procedure. Cryosurgery, often known as cryotherapy, or radiofrequency ablation, which includes administering heat, is another method for killing tumor cells.

Radiation Treatment

High-energy waves used in radiation treatment may be utilized to harm or kill cancer cells. This could prevent their growth and spread. Targeting cancer cells that can still exist after surgery is a common use of radiation. It is regarded as a local therapy, which means that it is often applied to a single location of the body.

Chemotherapy

A chemical medicinal treatment called chemotherapy is used to treat cancer. It affects the whole body and targets cancer cells that are developing quickly. If cancer has metastasized—that is, moved from the kidneys to other areas of the body—a doctor may advise it.

Immunotherapy

With the aid of immunotherapy, your body's immune system can more easily identify and combat cancerous cells. Pembrolizumab (Keytruda) and Nivolumab are two examples of immunotherapy used to treat kidney cancer (Opdivo).

Targeted Medicines

Targeted medications are designed to stop certain aberrant signals that kidney cancer cells emit. They may be able to prevent the growth of blood vessels that would otherwise feed the cancer cells with nutrition. Targeted medications include:

Sunitinib (Sunitinib), pazopanib (Votrient), lenvatinib (Lenvima), axitinib (Inlyta), and sorafenib (Nexavar) (Sutent)

Avoiding Kidney Cancer
The most effective strategy to lower your risk of kidney cancer is to lead a healthy lifestyle. You may take specific measures to lower your risk, such as:
- Not A Smoker
- keeping a healthy weight while eating a balanced diet
- regulating your blood pressure while protecting yourself from chemical contaminants at work

20. Cancer of the larynx
A kind of throat cancer that affects your larynx is called laryngeal cancer. Your voice box is called the larynx. It has muscles and cartilage that help you speak.

Your voice may suffer from this form of malignancy. If not treated right away, it might spread to other bodily areas.

4 percent of all malignancies in the US are head and neck cancers, according to the National Cancer Institute. The precise location of the tumor and the timing of the diagnosis both affect the survival rates.

Which signs and symptoms accompany laryngeal cancer?

The signs of laryngeal cancer are more noticeable than those of other forms of cancer. Among the most typical indications are:

- Squeaky voice
- Breathing problems
- Severe coughing, bloody cough, neck ache
- Throat and ear ache
- Eating difficulties neck swelling neck lumps
- An unexpected loss of weight

Who's susceptible to laryngeal cancer?

Your chance of acquiring laryngeal cancer is increased by certain lifestyle choices. These consist of:

- Smoking
- Smoking cigarettes
- Inadequate consumption of fruits and vegetables
- Large-scale use of processed food
- Consuming alcohol
- Asbestos contamination
- A history of throat cancer in the family

What laryngeal cancer therapies are available?

Your cancer stage will determine your course of treatment.

In the first phases of treatment, your doctor may choose to do surgery or radiation therapy. Surgery is often used to remove tumors. Cancer surgery has many risks. If cancer has had time to spread, they are more likely to happen. You could encounter:

Trouble breathing, swallowing, neck deformity, voice loss or alteration, permanently scarred neck

Radiation treatment then aims to eradicate any cancer cells that may still exist. Radiation treatment alone may be recommended by your doctor to treat minor malignancies.

Another kind of cancer treatment is chemotherapy. It can:

- Following radiation and surgery, eliminate any cancer cells that remain.
- Radiation therapy should be used to treat advanced cancer when surgery is not an option.
- Treating advanced cancer symptoms that can't be completely eradicated

Your doctor could suggest an alternative to surgery as the first course of therapy. Typically, this occurs when a tumor is tiny enough that no surgery is required. It could also happen if the operation is too late to be successful. Your quality of life should be preserved in any case.

Laryngeal cancer in its more advanced stages often has to be treated with a combination of surgery, radiation, and chemotherapy.

Substitute Treatments
You could find alternative treatments useful during laryngeal cancer therapy, including:
Yoga, meditation, acupuncture, and massage treatment

How May Laryngeal Cancer Be Avoided?
You may alter your lifestyle to lower your chance of laryngeal cancer by doing the following:

- Reduce or stop using tobacco in any way if you smoke.
- If you want to consume alcohol, do so sparingly.
- If at work you are exposed to asbestos or other poisons, use the appropriate protective gear.
- Maintain a healthy diet that includes foods high in antioxidants.

21. Leukemia Cancer

A malignancy of the blood cells is called leukemia. Red blood cells (RBCs), white blood cells (WBCs), and platelets are three of the major types of blood cells. Leukemia often refers to WBC malignancies.

WBCs play an important role in your immune system. Your body is shielded against invasion by them from: viruses, fungus, bacteria, aberrant cells and unfamiliar substances.

WBCs do not operate normally in leukemia. They may also divide excessively, ultimately displacing healthy cells.

WBCs are mostly created in the bone marrow, however, certain varieties may also be produced in the: lymph nodes, spleen, and thymus.

WBCs are generated and then move through the lymphatic and blood vessels of the body to combat infection in the tissues.

What signs or symptoms indicate leukemia?

Leukemia symptoms might include:

- Profuse perspiration, particularly at night (sometimes known as "night sweats")
- Unintentional weight loss weakness and exhaustion that does not improve with rest
- Bone soreness and sensitivity
- Swelling, painless lymph nodes (especially in the neck and armpits)
- Petechiae, or enlarged liver or spleen, are red skin lesions.
- Bruising and bleeding rapidly
- Cold or fever
- Frequent Infections

Organs that the cancer cells have invaded or impacted by leukemia might also exhibit symptoms. For instance, the following may occur if cancer spreads to the central nervous system: Headaches, nausea, dizziness, uncertainty, muscular control issues and seizures.

The kind and severity of leukemia determine how aggressively the disease spreads.

Leukemia may also expand to several bodily regions, such as the following:
lungs, digestive system, heart, kidneys, and testicles

Many Forms Of Leukemia

Leukemia may develop acutely (suddenly) or gradually over time (slow onset). The cancer cells proliferate swiftly in acute leukemia. The illness advances gradually in chronic leukemia, and the first symptoms may be relatively minor.

Additionally, leukemia is divided into groups based on the cells that are afflicted.

Myeloid leukemia, also known as **myelogenous leukemia,** is leukemia involving myeloid cells. The juvenile blood cells known as myeloid cells would typically grow into granulocytes or monocytes.

Lymphocytic leukemia is the name for leukemia that affects lymphocytes.

The four primary kinds of leukemia are as follows:

Myeloid leukemia, acute (AML)

Both children and adults may develop acute myeloid leukemia (AML). Around 20,000 new cases of AML are detected annually in the US, according to the Surveillance, Epidemiology, and End Results Program of the National Cancer Institute (NCI). The most common kind of leukemia is this one. For AML, the 5-year survival rate is 29.5%.

Leukemia acute lymphocytic (ALL)
Acute lymphocytic leukemia (ALL) typically affects young patients. According to the NCI, 6,000 new cases of ALL are suspected each year. The survival percentage for ALL after five years is 69.9%.

myeloid leukemia persistent (CML)
Most people with chronic myeloid leukemia (CML) are adults. The NCI estimates that 9,000 new cases of CML are diagnosed each year. The survival rate for CML after five years is 70.6%.

Leukemia chronic lymphocytic (CLL)

People over the age of 55 are more prone to develop chronic lymphocytic leukemia (CLL). Children seldom ever experience it. The NCI estimates that 21,000 new cases of CLL are diagnosed each year. The survival percentage for CLL after five years is 87.2%.

An extremely uncommon variant of CLL is called hairy cell leukemia. Its name is derived from how microscopic images of malignant cells look.

Dealing With Leukemia

Hematologist-oncologists often treat leukemia. These medical professionals are experts in cancer and blood conditions. The kind and stage of cancer determine the course of therapy. The patient's general health and other medical issues can have a role.

Some leukemia types develop gradually and might not need prompt treatment. However, one or more of the following is often used in leukemia treatment:

Chemotherapy: Drugs are used in chemotherapy to destroy leukemia cells. Depending on the kind of leukemia, you can take a single medication or a mix of many.

Radiation Treatment: High-energy radiation is used in radiation treatment to harm leukemia cells and stop their proliferation. You might get radiation in one place or all over your body.

Transplanting of stem cells: With a stem cell transplant, unhealthy bone marrow is replaced with healthy bone marrow from a donor or your own body (autologous transplantation) (called allogeneic transplantation). An alternative name for this treatment is a bone marrow transplant.

Biotherapy or immunotherapy: Treatments used in biological or immunotherapy assist your immune system in identifying and eliminating cancer cells.

Targeted treatment: The targeted treatment makes use of drugs that exploit weaknesses in cancer cells. Imatinib (Gleevec), for instance, is a targeted medication often used to treat CML.

22. Oral cancer

Cancer that appears in the tissues of the mouth or throat is referred to as oral cancer. It is a part of the wider category of tumors known as head and neck cancers. The squamous cells in your mouth, tongue, and lips are where the majority grow.

In the United States, there are more than 49,000 instances of oral cancer detected each year, with persons over 40 years old being the most often affected. The majority of the time, oral cancers are only found after they have migrated to the neck lymph nodes. The key to surviving oral cancer is early identification.

Oral Cancer Types.

Oral Cancers include: Lips, tongue, inner cheek, lining, gums, the floor of the mouth, and hard and soft palate.

Oral cancer symptoms are often initially identified by your dentist. By visiting the dentist every two years, you can keep your dentist informed about the condition of your mouth.

Signs and symptoms of Oral cancer

cancer symptoms include:

- A tumor or growth in your mouth, a sore on your lip or in your mouth that won't go away,
- Bleeding from your mouth, loose teeth, discomfort while swallowing, or difficulties wearing dentures.
- a persistent earache, a lump in your neck, or significant weight loss
- Numbness in the chin, neck, lower lip, or face
- Your mouth or lips have white, red, or red and white spots on them.
- throat irritation jaw ache or stiffness
- tongue ache.

Some of these signs, such as a sore throat or an earache, might be a sign of something else. Visit your dentist or doctor as soon as you can if you have any of these symptoms, particularly if they persist or you experience more than one at once.

Treatment Options For Oral Cancer

Depending on the kind, location, and stage of the disease upon diagnosis, many treatments are available for oral cancer.

Surgery

Surgery to remove the tumor and malignant lymph nodes is often the first line of treatment in the early stages. It's also possible to remove more tissue from the lips and neck.

Radiation Treatment

Another alternative is radiation treatment. For two to eight weeks, a doctor will direct radiation beams to the tumor once or twice per day, five days each week. Chemotherapy and radiation therapy are often used in the treatment of late stages.

Chemotherapy

Chemotherapy is a kind of medicine used to treat cancer. You may get the medication by mouth or via an intravenous line. Although some patients need to be hospitalized, the majority of patients get chemotherapy as outpatients.

Targeted treatment
Another kind of therapy is targeted therapy. Both the early and late stages of cancer may benefit from it. Drugs used in targeted treatment will attach to certain proteins on cancer cells and stop the proliferation of the cells.

Nutrition
A crucial component of your therapy for oral cancer is nutrition. Poor appetite and weight loss are frequent side effects of several medications that make it unpleasant or difficult to eat and swallow. Make sure to talk to your doctor about your diet.

You may create a meal that will be easy on your tongue and throat while still giving your body the calories, vitamins, and minerals it needs to recover by consulting a nutritionist.

Maintaining dental health

Finally, maintaining good oral health while receiving cancer therapy is an essential component of care. Maintain a moist mouth as well as clean teeth and gums.

23. Cancer Of The Lips

Lip lesions or tumors that are made of aberrant cells that proliferate uncontrollably give rise to lip cancer. One kind of oral cancer is lip cancer. Squamous cells are small, flat cells that line the: lips, mouth, tongue, cheeks throat, hard and soft palates etc.

Your chance of acquiring lip cancer may rise as a result of certain lifestyle decisions. These consist of:

- Smoking cigarettes.
- Excessive alcohol consumption.
- Excessive exposure to sun

Dentists are often the ones who first detect lip cancer symptoms, frequently during a regular dental examination. When caught early, lip cancer is largely treatable.

What Signs Are There Of Lip Cancer?
Lip cancer symptoms and signs include:
- A persistent ache, lesion, blister, ulcer, or lump in the mouth.
- A white or red spot on the lip
- Bruising or discomfort on the lips
- Inflammation of the jaw

Symptoms of lip cancer could be absent. Oftentimes, a normal dental examination is when a dentist first detects lip cancer. However, having a sore or lump on your lips does not always indicate that you have lip cancer. Any symptoms should be discussed with your dentist or doctor.

How is cancer of the lips treated?
Lip cancer may be treated with surgery, radiation therapy, and chemotherapy, to name a few.

Targeted therapy and experimental therapies like immunotherapy and gene therapy are further possibilities that could be considered.

The stage of the disease, how far it has advanced (including the size of the tumor), and your overall health all have a role in how it is treated, just like with other malignancies.

Surgery is often used to remove tiny tumors. This entails reconstructing the lip in addition to removing any cancerous tissue (cosmetically and functionally).

Radiation and chemotherapy may be used to decrease the tumor before or after surgery if it is bigger or has progressed to a later stage to lower the chance of recurrence.

Chemotherapy treatments disseminate medications throughout the body while lowering the likelihood of the disease returning or spreading.

For smokers, stopping before therapy may enhance the effectiveness of such treatment.

What can be done to avoid lip cancer?

Avoiding all forms of cigarette use, abstaining from excessive alcohol use, and minimizing exposure to both natural and artificial sunlight, especially tanning beds, are all ways to prevent lip cancer.

Dentists often make the first discovery of lip cancer patients. As a result, it's crucial to schedule frequent dental consultations with a qualified specialist, particularly if you're at a higher risk of developing lip cancer.

24. Ovarian Cancer

On each side of the uterus are two tiny, almond-shaped structures called the ovaries. The ovaries are where eggs are made. There are several locations on the ovary where ovarian cancer may develop.

In the ovary's germ, stromal, or epithelial cells, ovarian cancer may develop. The precursors of eggs are germ cells. The material of the ovary is made up of stromal cells. The outer layer of the ovary is made up of epithelial cells.

According to the American Cancer Society, there will be 22,240 new cases of ovarian cancer among women in the country in 2018, and 14,070 people will pass away from this disease. Women over the age of 63 accounts for around half of all instances.

Obvious Signs Of Ovarian Cancer

Ovarian cancer in its early stages can not show any signs. That might make it extremely difficult to find. However, some signs might be:

- Frequent bloating.
- Feeling full after a meal fast.
- Having trouble eating.
- A Frequent, urgent need to urination.
- Pain or discomfort in the pelvic or abdomen.

These signs appear out of the blue. They feel different from normal digestion and menstruating discomfort. They remain as well.

The following are other signs of ovarian cancer:
- Lower back pain.
- Discomfort during sexual activity.
- Constipation.
- Exhaustion.
- A change in the menstrual cycle.
- Weight gain, weight reduction, vaginal bleeding and acne.

You should visit a doctor if these symptoms persist for more than two weeks.

Ovarian Cancer Causes

Ovarian cancer is still poorly understood by researchers. The likelihood that a woman may get this form of cancer can be increased by a variety of risk factors, but these risk factors do not guarantee cancer development.

When cells in the body begin to grow and reproduce erratically, cancer develops. Researchers looking into ovarian cancer are attempting to pinpoint the specific genetic abnormalities that cause the illness.

These mutations may either be acquired or inherited from a parent. They thus happen throughout your lifespan.

Ovarian Cancer Types
Ovarian Epithelial Carcinoma
Ovarian cancer of the most prevalent form is epithelial cell carcinoma. It accounts for between 85% and 89 % of ovarian malignancies. It ranks as the fourth most frequent reason for cancer-related deaths in women.
Early on, this variety often shows no signs. Most patients don't get a diagnosis until the illness has progressed significantly.

Genetic Influences
Women who have a family history of any of the following are more likely to develop this kind of ovarian cancer:
- Breast cancer and ovarian cancer
- Ovarian cancer without breast cancer
- Colon cancer and ovarian cancer

The biggest risk group for ovarian cancer in women with two or more first-degree relatives who have the disease, such as a parent, sibling, or child. However, the risk rises if there is even one first-degree family who has the disease. Ovarian cancer risk is linked to the "breast cancer genes" BRCA1 and BRCA2.

Factors associated with higher survival
Epithelial ovarian cancer survivorship is connected to some variables, including:
- being younger having a well-differentiated tumor, or cancer cells that still closely resemble healthy cells.
- Early diagnosis
- having cancer caused by the BRCA1 and BRCA2 genes having a smaller tumor at the time of removal

Ovarian Germ Cell Cancer
The term "ovarian germ cell cancer" is used to refer to some distinct cancers. These malignancies arise from the egg-producing cells.

They often affect young girls and teenagers, with women in their 20s being the most susceptible.

These tumors have a propensity to spread widely and fast. Human chorionic gonadotropin is sometimes produced by tumors (HCG). A false-positive pregnancy test may result from this.

Most germ cell tumors may be effectively treated. The first course of therapy is surgery. After surgery, chemotherapy is strongly advised.

Ovarian stromal cell cancer

Ovarian cells give rise to stromal cell tumors. In addition to producing testosterone, progesterone, and estrogen, some of these cells also generate ovarian hormones.

Ovarian stromal cell tumors are uncommon and progress slowly. They exude testosterone and estrogen. Acne and facial hair development may be brought on by too much testosterone. Uterine hemorrhage may result from an excess of estrogen. These signs might be fairly obvious.

As a result, stromal cell cancer is more likely to be found early on. The prognosis for those with stromal cell carcinoma is often favorable. Typically, surgery is used to treat this kind of cancer.

Cancer of the ovary treatment

The kind, stage, and whether you want to have children in the future will all affect how your ovarian cancer is treated.

Surgery.

Surgery may be used to assess the cancer's stage, confirm the diagnosis, and perhaps even eliminate the tumor.

Your surgeon will attempt to remove all cancerous tissue during surgery. To determine if cancer has spread, they could also take a sample. Whether or not you want to get pregnant in the future may influence how extensive the operation is.

If you have stage 1 cancer and want to get pregnant in the future, surgical options include:

- Surgical excision of the cancerous ovary and ovarian biopsy.
- Excision of the omentum, or fatty tissue, that is linked to certain abdominal organs.
- Elimination of the pelvic and abdominal lymph nodes.
- Abdominal fluid buildup and biopsies of other tissues.

Surgery For Advanced Ovarian Cancer

If you don't want to have kids, surgery is more involved. If your cancer is in stages 2, 3, or 4, you could potentially need further surgery. It's possible that having all cancerous tissue completely removed will keep you from becoming pregnant in the future. This comprises:

- Elimination of the uterus.
- Removal of the fallopian tubes and ovaries.
- Taking out the omentum.
- EXCISION of as much cancer-containing tissue as feasible.
- Biopsy of any potential malignant tissue.

Surgery is often followed by chemotherapy. Both intravenous and abdominal administration of medications are options. This is referred to as **intraperitoneal therapy.** Chemotherapy side effects might include: hair loss, vomiting, exhaustion, and difficulty sleeping

Therapy For Symptoms

You may need further therapy for the symptoms the cancer is causing while your doctor gets ready to treat or remove the malignancy. Ovarian cancer patients often experience pain.

Organs, muscles, nerves, and bones adjacent may experience pressure from the tumor. The discomfort may be more severe depending on the size of the malignancy.

Pain might potentially be a side effect of therapy. You may have pain and suffering as a result of surgery, radiation, and chemotherapy.

Ovarian Cancer: Is It Preventable?

Early signs of ovarian cancer are quite uncommon. As a consequence, it often doesn't become apparent until it has gone into advanced stages. Ovarian cancer cannot presently be prevented, but there are things you may do to reduce your chance of getting it.

These elements consist of:

- Using contraceptive tablets
- Nursing after giving birth
- hysterectomy tubal ligation (commonly known as "getting your tubes tied")

Hysterectomy and tubal ligation should only be carried out when necessary. Lowering your risk of ovarian cancer may be a legitimate medical justification for some. However, you should first go through other preventative measures with your doctor.

If you have ovarian cancer in your family, you should speak with your doctor about early screening. Some DNA alterations may increase your chance of developing ovarian cancer in the future. Both you and your doctor may be more alert to changes if you are aware of whether you have certain mutations.

25. Pancreatic cancer

The pancreas, a crucial endocrine organ situated beneath the stomach, develops pancreatic cancer in its tissues. By manufacturing the digestive enzymes that the body requires to break down fats, carbs, and proteins, the pancreas plays a crucial role in digestion.

Glucagon and insulin are two more crucial hormones that the pancreas generates. The regulation of the metabolism of glucose (sugar) is carried out by these hormones. When glucose levels are too low, glucagon helps boost them. Insulin aids in the metabolism of glucose by cells to produce energy.

Due to the pancreas' location, pancreatic cancer may be difficult to detect and is often found at a later stage of the illness.
According to the American Cancer Society, pancreatic cancer accounts for 7% of cancer fatalities and roughly 3% of cancer diagnoses in the country.

According to the kind of cell they originate in, there are two primary forms of pancreatic cancer:

Cancer of the pancreas: The most common kind of pancreatic cancer is this one. Exocrine cells, which produce digestive enzymes, are where it all begins.

Neuroendocrine Tumors Of The Pancreas: The endocrine cells, which produce hormones that have an impact on everything from mood to metabolism, are where this less common kind of pancreatic cancer begins.

Signs Of Pancreatic Cancer

Before it has progressed to an advanced stage, pancreatic cancer often shows no signs. As a consequence, pancreatic cancer often has no early symptoms.

Some of the most typical pancreatic cancer symptoms might be modest, even at more advanced stages.

Pancreatic cancer may develop the following symptoms as it advances:

- Reduced appetite.
- Unintended loss of weight.
- Back pain that may also be present with your stomach ache.
- A lower back ache.
- Clots of blood (often in the leg, which can cause redness, pain, and swelling).
- Jaundice (yellowing skin and eyes) (yellowing skin and eyes).
- Depression.
- Greasy or pale-colored stools.
- Brown or dark urine.
- Rough skin.
- Nausea/vomiting.

Your blood sugar levels may be affected by pancreatic cancer. This may sometimes result in diabetes (or the worsening of preexisting diabetes).

Remember that the symptoms mentioned above might be brought on by some less significant medical issues.

Causes Of Pancreatic Cancer

There is no known cause of pancreatic cancer.

It is unknown why aberrant cells start to proliferate and form tumors within the pancreas, which is how pancreatic cancer develops.

Normal cell growth and cell death occur in small quantities. An increase in the generation of aberrant cells is seen in cases of cancer. Over time, these cells replace healthy ones.

There is no known primary cause of pancreatic cancer, although some risk factors may make you more likely to have it.

These consist of:

- **Using Tobacco**: Smoking may be responsible for 20 to 35 percent of occurrences of pancreatic cancer.
- **Excessive Alcohol Use**: Three or more alcoholic beverages each day might make you more vulnerable. Another risk factor for pancreatitis is alcohol use.

Pancreatitis is inherited and chronic: The effect of excessive drinking over an extended period is often chronic pancreatitis. Additionally, pancreatitis may run in families.

Weight: Obesity or being overweight, especially in early adulthood, may make you more at risk.

Diet: Although specialists are still trying to determine the precise relationship between dietary components and pancreatic cancer risk, eating a diet heavy in red and processed meats, fried foods, sweets, or cholesterol may raise your risk.

Sex: Men are somewhat more likely than women to acquire pancreatic cancer.

Exposed at work: Up to 12% of occurrences of pancreatic cancer may be related to working with specific chemicals, especially those used in metalworking and insecticides.

Age: Pancreatic cancer diagnoses are more common in patients between the ages of 65 and 74.

Diabetes: If you have type 1 or type 2 diabetes, your chance of getting pancreatic cancer may be greater.

Race: Black individuals in the US have the highest incidence of pancreatic cancer. There is still a need for greater research into the underlying reasons for racial differences in pancreatic cancer rates, according to experts. Research from 2018 reveals this is caused by a combination of lifestyle, socioeconomic, and genetic variables.

Family background: Around 10% of those who develop pancreatic cancer have a family history of the disease.

Infections: Although the precise connection between H. pylori infection and pancreatic cancer is unclear, having a history of the illness in your digestive system may raise your risk. Additionally, having hepatitis B might raise your risk by up to 24 percent.

Your chance of developing pancreatic cancer may be increased by certain genetic alterations and mutations. These conditions include, among others:

- Syndrome of Peutz-Jeghers.
- Hereditary breast and ovarian cancer syndrome.
- Lynch syndrome.
- Familial atypical multiple mole melanoma syndromes.
- Inherited pancreatitis.

Treatment For Pancreatic Cancer

Killing malignant cells and halting the progression of the disease are the two basic objectives of treatment for pancreatic cancer. Depending on the stage of cancer, the best treatment plan will be determined.

The primary forms of therapy are:

Surgery: Parts of the pancreas are removed during surgery to treat pancreatic cancer. This can get rid of the initial tumor, but it won't get rid of cancer that has spread to other places. Therefore, surgery is often not advised for pancreatic cancer in its late stages.

Radiation treatment: To destroy cancer cells, high-energy beams such as X-rays are utilized.

Chemotherapy: Anticancer medications are used to eradicate cancer cells and aid in halting their further development.

Targeted treatment: Drugs and antibodies are used to specifically target cancer cells, avoiding the damage that chemotherapy and radiation treatment might cause to healthy cells.

Immunotherapy. Your immune system is stimulated in a variety of ways to attack the malignancy.
A doctor could advise combining several treatment approaches in specific circumstances. For instance, chemotherapy may be administered before surgery.

Treatment options for pancreatic cancer in the late stages may put more emphasis on symptom control and pain management.

Prevention Of Pancreatic Cancer

There is now no effective technique to prevent pancreatic cancer since its exact etiology is still unknown.

Some of these factors, such as your family history and age, cannot be altered even if they may raise your chance of getting pancreatic cancer.

However, making a few lifestyle adjustments might lower your risk:

1. Quit smoking: If you presently smoke, research several methods to support your efforts to stop.

2. Limit alcohol consumption to lower your chance of developing pancreatic cancer and chronic pancreatitis.

3. Maintain a healthy weight: Overweight and obesity may result from a variety of

circumstances, some of which are beyond your control. If you are obese or overweight, you may want to discuss maintaining a healthy weight with a medical expert.

4. Include whole foods in your diet. Red meat, processed meat, sweets, and fried meals are some examples of foods that may raise your risk of pancreatic cancer. You don't have to eliminate them from your diet, but you should try to balance them out with lean meats, nutritious grains, and fresh or frozen fruits and vegetables.

Consult a healthcare provider as soon as you can if you're exhibiting symptoms that you believe might be related to pancreatic cancer, particularly if you're at higher risk for the disease. Although many illnesses might present with the same symptoms, pancreatic cancer responds best to therapy when discovered in its earliest stages.

26. Skin cancer

The most prevalent kind of cancer is skin cancer. It happens when skin cells develop in an uncontrolled manner. Doctors may also determine the kind of skin cancer by looking at the cells.

Understanding skin cancer's many kinds and how they impact the body is the greatest method to comprehend it.

Skin Cancer Types
Base Cell Cancer

Basal cells, which are skin cells that replace older ones in the lowest layer of the epidermis, are where basal cell cancer starts. This kind of skin cancer often develops on the skin's surface.

Basal cell carcinoma often doesn't spread to other body parts. When it happens, it may even pose a life-threatening situation.

Around 80% of all skin malignancies are basal cell tumors, according to the American Cancer Society (ACS).

Cancerous Squamous Cells

The cells on the outermost layer of the epidermis are impacted by squamous cell carcinoma.

Squamous cells are also seen in tissues including the mucous membranes and lungs. The term "cutaneous squamous cell cancer" refers to squamous cell cancer that develops in the skin.

Those parts of the body that are regularly exposed to ultraviolet (UV) rays are where this form of cancer is most usually detected. Although it is a relatively curable disorder, going untreated increases the risk of death.

Squamous cell carcinoma is the second most prevalent kind of skin cancer, according to the Skin Cancer Foundation.

The American Carcinoma Society (ACS) estimates that 5.4 million cases of basal and squamous cell cancer are diagnosed annually. Your head and neck are two locations of your body where they are most prone to appear.

Melanoma

Melanoma, which makes up 1% of all skin cancers, is a different type of skin cancer. The cells that provide your skin pigment give rise to this form of cancer. Melanocytes are the name for these cells. Melanocytes produce benign moles that have the potential to develop into a malignancy.

Your body may grow melanomas everywhere. In males, the chest and back are more often affected, but in women, the legs are.

When detected early, most melanomas may be treated. But if left untreated, they could spread to other areas of your body and become more difficult to cure. Additionally, compared to basal and squamous cell skin tumors, melanomas have a higher propensity to spread.

Skin cancer with Merkel cells

An uncommon kind of skin cancer known as Merkel cell skin cancer is brought on by an overabundance of Merkel cells. A 2019 study identified Merkel cells as a specific subset of epidermal cells.

According to an analysis from 2021, there are around 1,500 instances of Merkel cell cancer reported each year in the US. It seems to affect males more often than women, and white individuals more often.

Despite being rare, it may swiftly spread to other bodily areas, making it very deadly.

Skin-related lymphoma

White blood cells in the body function as an aspect of the immune system to protect against illness and infection. Lymphocytes are another name for these cells.

Skin lymphoma is the term for when cells on the skin begin to proliferate erratically. It is sometimes referred to as cutaneous lymphoma, according to the ACS.

The Kaposi sarcoma

On the skin, Kaposi sarcoma (KS) tumors or patches might be red, brown, or purple. Lesions is another name for the regions.

KS lesions often show up on the face, foot, or legs. Additionally, lesions may develop in the mouth, lymph nodes, or vaginal region. You may not feel any symptoms if they stay on the surface.

However, KS lesions may spread internally, for example to the stomach or esophagus. They risk becoming fatal when they do this because bleeding might result.

The actin keratosis

These are often little areas of skin that are red, pink, or brown. Despite not being malignant, they are regarded as a kind of precancer. These skin lesions might turn into squamous cell carcinoma if left untreated.

Skin cancer signs and symptoms

Because no two skin tumors are the same, some may not exhibit many early signs. Nevertheless, abnormal changes to your skin may be an indication of several cancers. Being aware of changes in your skin might speed up the diagnosing process.

Keep an eye out for warning symptoms of skin cancer, such as

- Skin Conditions: The appearance of a fresh mole, an odd growth, a lump, a sore, a scaly patch, or a dark area that doesn't go away.
- Asymmetry: A lesion or mole doesn't have two identical halves.
- Border. The margins of lesions are rough and irregular.
- Color: A distinctive hue, such as white, pink, black, blue, or red, characterizes a spot. Additionally, a lesion could have more than one color.
- Diameter: A pencil eraser would be a good comparison for the size, which is greater than 1/4 inch.
- Evolving: You can tell whether a mole has changed by looking at its size, shape, color, or any accompanying symptoms like itchiness, discomfort, or bleeding.

If you suspect a lesion on your skin could be skin cancer, it's vital to be aware of all the warning signals that might be present.

Skin cancer causes and risk factors.

Skin cancer develops when your skin cells' DNA undergoes alterations. These mutations lead to uncontrolled growth and the formation of a mass of cancerous skin cells.

There are several unidentified causes of skin cancer. Researchers are unsure of why some moles develop into melanomas whereas the majority do not.

Risk factors, however, may increase your vulnerability to skin malignancies like melanoma.

UV radiation exposure

According to the Centers for Disease Control and Prevention (CDC), exposure to UV radiation increases the chance of developing several different forms of skin cancer. UV radiation exposure may be caused by: the tanning bed, solar rays

Your skin cells become damaged by UV radiation. Skin cancer arises when the injury results in excessive cell proliferation.

Moles: As was previously indicated, moles are not usually a sign of skin cancer. However, if you have a lot of them, they have a higher chance of turning into melanoma.

Light hair, complexion, and freckles
People with lighter skin have a higher chance of developing skin cancer, particularly if they have:

- Natural green or blue eyes,
- red or blonde hair,
- fair skin that is prone to sunburn or freckles

Relatives With Skin Cancer
You are at greater risk if your parents, siblings, or children are diagnosed with melanoma, according to Cancer Research UK. According to 2015 research, this could be caused by a shared sun-loving lifestyle, having fair skin, or familial genetic variations.
- If skin cancer runs in your family, specialists advise you to:

- Self-skin checks should be done once each month.
- Use sunscreen and other sun protection measures first.
- Avoid sun exposure and use tanning beds.
- Visit your dermatologist often to get your skin examined.

Prior Skin Cancer History

The likelihood of developing skin cancer again is increased if you've already had it.

In a 2018 research of 969 skin cancer patients, it was shown that 17% of them went on to acquire recurrent skin cancer, particularly if they were older individuals. The startling figure emphasizes the need for regular follow-up appointments with your doctor to carefully track any recurrence.

The next time, it can even be a different kind of skin cancer. For instance, your risk of developing melanoma increases if you've had squamous cell skin cancer.

Compromised Immune System

Your risk of developing skin cancer increases when other illnesses or medical procedures weaken your immune system.

If any of the following applies to you:

- The use of chemotherapy.
- Have an autoimmune condition that results in a compromised immune system.
- Take certain drugs

Old age

Although skin cancer may occur in adolescents and young adults, it most often affects those over the age of 30.

Skin Cancer Remedies

Various variables will affect the suggested course of therapy for you. These include cancers like: size, location, type, stage.

Your healthcare team may suggest one or more of the following procedures after taking these variables into account:

Cryosurgery: The tissue is destroyed when the growth thaws after being frozen with liquid nitrogen.

Amputation Surgery: The doctor removes the tumor along with some nearby good skin.

Mohs procedure: Throughout this process, the growth is stripped away layer by layer. A microscope is used to inspect each layer until no irregular cells are left.

Both electrodesiccation and curettage: The cancerous cells are removed with a large spoon-shaped blade, and any leftover cells are then burned by an electric needle.

Chemotherapy: To eliminate the cancer cells, this medication may be ingested, administered topically, or injected intravenously (IV).
Photodynamic treatment Drugs and laser light both kill cancer cells.
Radiation: The cancer cells are destroyed by intense energy beams.

Biological Treatment: The immune system is boosted by biological therapies to combat cancer cells.

Immunotherapy: The immune system is boosted by medications so that it can eliminate cancer cells.

Self-exams for skin cancer

Some skin cancer warning symptoms may be seen by someone without medical knowledge. A mirror and a strategy for checking yourself at least once a month is all you need.

Use a full-length mirror and do it in a well-lit area for the best effects. A portable mirror is quite useful for those challenging to view regions. A loved one might also be enlisted to ensure that no detail is overlooked.

Take your time and pay attention to any freckles, mole patterns, or other skin imperfections. When you get your monthly checks, inspect them for any changes. Bleeding and slowly healing wounds are examples of changes. Inform your doctor if you see any potential problem areas.

To ensure you don't miss a lot, the ACS suggests that you do the following actions:

- Check your: face, ears, neck, chest, stomach, and breasts while facing the mirror.
- As you turn to your arms, elevate them to inspect your armpits.
- Inspect the palms and tops of your hands.
- Observe the fingernails and fingers.
- Examine your thighs, front and back shins, front and back feet, top and bottom toes, and toenails while seated.
- Examine your buttocks, vaginal region, lower and upper back, back of neck, and ears with a hand mirror.
- Finally, examine your scalp with a comb.

Preventing Skin Cancer

Avoid leaving your skin exposed to UV rays from the sun and other sources for long periods to reduce your chance of developing skin cancer. For instance:

Avoid Using Sunlamps And Tanning Beds.

By remaining indoors or in the shade from 10 a.m. to 4 p.m., when the sun is at its heaviest, you may avoid direct sun exposure.

At least 30 minutes before going outside, use sunscreen and lip balm with an SPF of 30 or higher to any exposed skin, and reapply as necessary.

When you're outdoors during the day, dress in dry, dark, tightly woven clothing with a broad brim.

Don't forget to protect yourself from UVB and UVA rays by wearing sunglasses.

Additionally, it's crucial to periodically check your skin for changes like patches or new growths. If you see anything unusual, let your doctor know.

Early detection and treatment of skin cancer may help you have a better prognosis in the long run.

27. Melanoma Cancer.

Skin cancer known as melanoma develops when malignant cells begin to proliferate in melanocytes, or cells that create melanin. These are the cells in charge of coloring the skin. Even in the eyes, melanoma may develop anywhere on the skin. Despite the rarity of the disorder, more individuals are now receiving melanoma diagnoses than ever before.

Symptoms include:
- an unevenly shaped mole or mark on the asymmetrical skin. The borders could seem scalloped or notched.
- a mole or blemish with several hues (rather than being all one shade of brown or black). Brown, black, white, red, pink, or even blue melanoma are all possible.
- a red, white, or blue mole or mark
- a mole that is bigger than a pencil eraser's tip
- a mole or mark that is expanding rapidly, has altered in color or form, or both
- bleeding, itchy, or crusting mole or spot

Experts advise checking your skin from head to toe once a month for any possible indications of skin cancer and having your doctor examine your skin once a year as well since melanoma creates obvious changes on your skin.

Melanoma Prevention Methods

Melanoma is an uncommon kind of skin cancer, as was previously established. Sometimes a person might get melanoma despite not having a long history of sun exposure. This can be because the condition runs in the family. You may yet take the following actions to lessen your chance of developing melanoma:

- To protect yourself from the sun's rays, limit your time spent in the sun and seek out shelter whenever you can.

- Avoid trying to get a tan by using sunlamps or tanning beds. The American Cancer Society claims that those who use tanning beds have a higher chance of developing melanoma.

- Remember to slide on a shirt, slop on sunscreen, slap on a hat, and wrap on sunglasses to shield your eyes from the sun by using the mnemonic method "Slip! Slop! Slap... and Wrap!"

Check your skin often for any indications that a mole is changing. Some individuals may take monthly photos of their skin and compare them to see if any changes have occurred.

Any time a person notices a mole that is changing or a patch of skin that looks crusted, cracked, or otherwise ulcerated should be examined by a dermatologist to rule out the possibility of a malignant lesion.

28. Vulvar Cancer

When aberrant tissue cells proliferate uncontrolled, vulvar cancer develops. Cancer may appear everywhere in the body, and depending on the kind and where it is located, both the symptoms and the course of therapy will vary. The female reproductive system may be impacted by some cancers, including vulvar carcinoma.

A female's external genitalia, or vulva, may develop cancer. The vagina's inner and outer lips, the clitoris, and the introitus, or entrance, are all considered to be parts of the vulva. The vulva also includes the glands that are close to the vaginal entrance. Other areas of the vulva may also be impacted, particularly if the disease becomes larger. Vulvar cancer often affects the outer lips of the vagina.

Which Signs and Symptoms Indicate Vulvar Cancer?

Vulvar carcinoma may be undetected in its early stages. When symptoms do materialize, they may comprise:

- Uncommon bleeding
- Itching in the vulvar area
- A discolored region of skin that hurts while urinating and is painful around the vulvar area
- lump or sores that resemble warts on the vulva

Who Has a Chance of Getting Vulvar Cancer?

Vulvar cancer has some risk factors, yet the specific etiology of the disease is unknown. These consist of:

- Being over 55 and smoking.
- Vulvar intraepithelial neoplasia is present.
- Having AIDS or the HIV
- Having an infection with the human papillomavirus (HPV).
- A background of genital warts.
- Having a skin disease like lichen planus that may damage the vulva.

The Staging of Vulvar Cancer

Your doctor may categorize cancer's severity using staging. This enables them to design a successful treatment strategy for you. The original tumor's location, whether the disease has spread to neighboring lymph nodes, the size and number of tumors, and their number are also considerations during staging.

Vulvar cancer commonly has stages 0 through 4. The harshness increases as the stage rise:

Stage 0

Very early cancer that is limited to the vulva's surface is referred to as stage 0 cancer.

Stage 1

Just the vulva or the perineum are affected by stage 1 malignancy. The skin between the vaginal entrance and the anus is known as the perineum. The lymph nodes or other parts of the body have not been invaded by the tumor.

Stage 2

The lower sections of the urethra, vagina, and anus are among the surrounding sites where stage 2 cancer has progressed from the vulva.

Stage 3

Lymph nodes close by have been affected by stage 3 cancer.

Stage 4

The lymph nodes, higher sections of the urethra, or vagina have more widely disseminated stage 4A cancer. In other instances, the pelvic bone, rectum, or bladder have been affected by the tumors.

Cancer in stage 4B has metastasized to distant organs or lymph nodes.

Treatment Options for Vulvar Cancer

Depending on the stage of your cancer, your treatment strategy will vary. Four different types of standard treatments exist, though:

Use of lasers

To kill cancer cells, laser therapy uses intense light. To target and eliminate the tumors, the light beams pass through a tiny tube known as an endoscope. When compared to other treatments, laser therapy typically results in less bleeding and scarring. Often, it can be done as an outpatient procedure, allowing you to leave the hospital the same day as your treatment.

Surgery

The most frequently used therapy for vulvar cancer is surgery. Surgery can be done in a wide variety of ways. The type of surgery you receive will depend on the cancer's stage and your general health.

Cuts made locally

If cancer hasn't spread to nearby nodes or organs, a local excision might be performed. The procedure entails removing the affected area and a small amount of the surrounding healthy tissue. Additionally, lymph nodes may be removed.

Vulvectomy

A vulvectomy is an additional surgical choice. Your doctor will either perform a radical vulvectomy or a partial vulvectomy during this procedure, depending on how much of the vulva is removed.

Penetration of the Pelvis

Pelvic exenteration may be done in cases of advanced or severe vulvar cancer. Your surgeon might take out the: depending on where cancer has spread to.

Lower colon and vagina

ovaries, rectum, bladder, and vulva

Your surgeon will make a stoma after removing your bladder, rectum, and colon to allow your feces and urine to exit your body.

Radiological Therapy

High-energy radiation is used in radiation therapy to shrink tumors and kill cancer cells. This type of treatment can be delivered externally, which means a machine will direct the rays to the cancerous area. In other circumstances, radioactive seeds or wires may be inserted to administer radiation therapy internally.

Chemotherapy

Chemotherapy is a potent form of chemical drug therapy that works to slow or stop the growth of cancer cells. When cancer has spread to other body organs and is more advanced, it is the preferred course of treatment. You can administer the medication intravenously or orally depending on the kind of medication being given. Additionally, a topical cream is available.

29. Cancer of the appendix.

Near the start of your big intestines, your appendix links to your colon in the form of a small tube-shaped sac. Although its function is still unknown, some researchers believe that your appendix could be a component of your immune system.

Appendiceal carcinoma is another name for appendix cancer. It happens when normally behaving cells develop aberrant growth patterns. After the appendix has been surgically removed, these malignant cells form a lump or tumor within the organ, which is often discovered by mistake.

What are the causes of appendix cancer?

No preventable risk factors have been found, and the etiology of appendix cancer is mostly unclear. However, appendix cancer is uncommon in youngsters and grows more prevalent as people age.

How to treat appendix cancer?

The following factors determine how to treat appendix cancer: Type of tumor, stage of the malignancy, and general health of the patient.

Throughout your treatment, a diverse team of medical experts will assist you. A wide range of experts will be on your team, including physicians, nurse practitioners, nutritionists, counselors, and others. Your cancer will be surgically removed by a specialist known as a surgical oncologist, and your chemotherapy regimen will be created by a medical oncologist.

Surgery

The most popular form of therapy for locally advanced appendix cancer is surgery. The appendix is often removed as part of therapy if the cancer is solely present in the appendix. Another name for this is appendectomy.

Your doctor can advise removing half of your colon as well as certain lymph nodes if you have certain forms of appendix cancer or if the tumor is bigger. Hemicolectomia are operations that include removing half of the colon.

Your doctor could advise cytoreductive surgery, also known as debulking if cancer has spread. The surgeon will do this sort of surgery to remove the tumor, any surrounding fluid, and maybe any associated neighboring organs.

Chemotherapy

If the tumor is more than 2 cm in size, chemotherapy may be used either before or after surgery.

In particular, the lymph nodes have seen the spread of the malignancy and if the cancer is aggressive.

Systemic chemotherapy administered intravenously or orally is one kind of chemotherapy.

- Regional chemotherapy that is administered directly into the abdomen includes EPIC (intraperitoneal chemotherapy) and HIPEC (hyperthermic intraperitoneal chemotherapy), which combine systemic and regional chemotherapies.

Radiation Treatment

Appendix cancer is seldom treated with radiation treatment. It could be advised, however, if your cancer spreads to other bodily areas.

Imaging Exams.

Following surgery, your doctor will order imaging exams like a CT scan or MRI scan to ascertain whether the tumor is gone.